UNDERSTANDING A WOMAN'S DEPRESSION

Understanding a

BRENDA

Woman's Depression

POINSETT

Tyndale House
Publishers, Inc.
Wheaton, Illinois

ACKNOWLEDGMENTS
Two doctors helped me immensely in recognizing and getting over my own depression and in the preparation of this manuscript. I'm grateful for the personal help and technical assistance given to me by Dr. Michael G. Lundy and Dr. Michael D. Dubriwny.

I'm also grateful to friends and acquaintances who have allowed me to share portions of their struggle with depression. These people are mentioned by first name within the manuscript, and, in some of the cases, the names have been changed.

All Scripture references are from the *King James Version* of the Bible unless otherwise indicated.

First printing, April 1984
Library of Congress Catalog Card Number 83–51595
ISBN 0-8423-7764-6, paper

Printed in the United States of America

To

CARILEEN

who never stopped calling

CONTENTS

ONE
WHAT DEPRESSION IS

Have you ever made an insignificant comment, only to look back later and wonder at your naiveté?

"I never get depressed," I boldly proclaimed to a friend of mine as our families were having dinner together one evening. Now, looking back, I can only wonder at the comment. At the time, my husband was "in between jobs." Just a month earlier, Bob had been fired from a job he dearly loved, one to which we both felt God had called him. A little over a year before that, Bob had been fired from another job. So within eighteen months, Bob had lost two jobs.

At the time, Bob was working at a window factory for minimum wage, trying to earn enough to buy gas and groceries for our family of five. We were trying to stretch Bob's severance pay to cover house payments and utilities until he could find another job.

Financial worries, disappointment in God's leadership, and job losses (even if they are the spouse's job) are the kinds of things which make people depressed. But I was not depressed and hadn't been, through both firings.

I attributed my lack of depression to a strong daily devotional life of prayer and Bible study. "Whatever comes my way, whatever gets me down, once I have my devotional time in the morning, I'm ready to go again," I said.

But now, *three* depressions later, I can only look back on my comment as a naive one. It was naive in many ways. I had no idea how I, as a woman, could hurt over what happened to my husband. Neither did I realize the power our subconscious mind can have over us, nor what destruction repressed feelings can cause. I was surprised to learn that even spiritual resources such as prayer and Bible reading can lose their effectiveness if the will is not engaged. In addition to these things, I simply didn't know what depression was. I was aware of depressive feelings, but I did not know there was such a thing as an illness called depression. I had a lot to learn.

WHAT DEPRESSION IS

Depression is a vague term used to describe many different things. Depression can be a mood, a symptom of an illness, or an illness in itself.

Many of us talk about "being depressed" at different times. We use the words lightly to indicate a passing mood. A down feeling. The blahs. Feeling blue. We may say we're depressed when we need a permanent or when our car breaks down three times in one week.

> We all go around using expressions like, "I'm depressed," or "It's depressing," to cover a hundred different feelings that we haven't bothered to sort out. We may be miserable, unhappy, disappointed, disillusioned, bitter, desperate, despairing, disconsolate, downhearted, grieving, downtrodden, exploited, distraught, frustrated, dispirited, fed up, or simply tired.[1]

For those times when we don't feel good about life and we are down on ourselves, we call the mood depression.

Many things can make us feel down. We feel down after suffering emotional or physical stress, particularly when we are tired. The weather affects our mood. The time of year affects our mood. Some people experience down feelings during the Christmas season or in the spring of the year. The economic climate of the country affects our feelings, and so can a host of other things.

These moods fluctuate in intensity and in length, depending upon the conditions involved. When we get that permanent, when the car gets repaired, or when Christmas is over, we are going to feel better. The key is *temporary.* The bad mood is there, but it will pass.

A down mood may also be experienced when something is physically wrong. Depressive feelings may be a symptom of a physical illness or disorder. Depressive feelings often accompany viral illnesses, or even a minor infection. Body disorders which list depression as a symptom include ulcers, rheumatoid arthritis, hypoglycemia, hypothyroidism, and fatigue.

Along the same line, depression may emerge as a side effect of some kinds of drugs or medication. For example, reserpine, a treatment for high blood pressure, brings about depression in 15 percent of the people using it. The same low kind of feelings described as a depressive mood may be present, and they may persist longer. When the physical problem is cleared up, the depressive feelings go away.

In addition to being a mood or a symptom of an illness, depression may also be an illness in itself. When I made my comment about never getting depressed, I didn't know there was an illness called depression. Known as clinical depression, it's a disorder that includes both physical and psychological symptoms.

Clinical depression is a bad mood that persists and persists. It doesn't leave when Christmas is over or when the physical difficulty is cleared up. It stays and stays, making itself at home, until it permeates our nature. When it does, we lose our ability to cope and to manage life as it is. Life becomes an ongoing struggle characterized by sadness, hopelessness, and despair.

The person with clinical depression undergoes changes. The once-talkative woman becomes silent and withdrawn. The woman who enjoys cooking *and eating* starts losing weight, noticeably so. When her friends ask her what her dieting secret is, she shrugs her shoulders and says, "I just don't feel like eating."

Furthermore, the changes persist. The loss of interest in conversation or food may continue for months. There may be other changes—a change in sleeping patterns or sexual desire. With the changes comes a morbid drop in confidence. She sees no way of improving her situation.

The most frequent way depression is described is, "I feel like I'm down in a well and can't get out." To that description, I would add, "The well has very slippery walls." Once in the well, it's very difficult to get out, for every attempt made involves sliding back several times.

One woman described depression as a live being. "For me, depression is a monster—maybe a demon, who knows?" she said. "He has a distinctive personality; he's seductive and sinister in nature. He made his way into my life without my inviting him in. He mocks my every action. With his long arms, he wraps himself around and around me until I feel like I'll never be free of him again."

Clinical depression is painful. It hurts, and the pain is as real as any form of physical pain. "Many persons who have experienced both severe physical and emotional pain have stated emphatically that emotional pain is worse than physical pain. They would prefer broken bones to a broken heart!"[2]

Clinical depression is more severe and longer lasting than a low mood. It is different from other illnesses that have depression as a symptom. It is an illness within itself, with clear-cut symptoms of its own. These symptoms are both psychological and physical. This book is going to be concerned primarily with clinical depression, which from this point on, we'll simply call depression. However, the women who experience depressive moods will also find this book helpful. The two—depressive moods and depressive illnesses—are closely related. What we learn about one will help us deal with the other one.

WHAT DEPRESSION IS NOT

To further our understanding of depression, we need to consider what depression is not. Depression is often confused with anxiety, loneliness, grief, and sadness. How do these emotions differ from depression?

Anxiety is an important part of our biological alarm system. It alerts us to the presence of threat or danger. Anxiety signals the existence of a problem which will require some action on our part. Too much anxiety is not good for us; it can put our physical and mental resources under strain. But not feeling any anxiety would represent a greater danger.

Some experts refer to anxiety as a "biological call to battle." In contrast, depression is "after the battle is over."

> . . . when one is feeling highly anxious, the inner urges are toward taking action, doing something, solving some problem, trying to identify and to deal with whatever it is that one *experiences* as threatening. But the person who is depressed is dominated by other feelings—by feelings of hopelessness, helplessness, worthlessness and the impulse to take no action because nothing can help and the problems are insoluble in any case . . . .[3]

Anxiety says, "We've got a problem; let's do something." Depression says, "We're defeated; there's nothing we can do."

Just as depression is not the same thing as anxiety, neither is it the same thing as loneliness. In true loneliness, as distressing as it is, there is a drive within to end the loneliness. A new relationship is attempted. A lost relationship is mended. Even a shy person will make what is for her gallant efforts to end her loneliness.

Depressed people do experience lonely feelings. Almost all of them complain of no one caring about them. The difference is, the people who are only lonely reach out to end their loneliness. The depressed person succumbs to her lonely feelings. She gives up hope of finding any satisfactory relationships. She surrenders to her isolation. "If I called someone, she probably wouldn't be at home, or she wouldn't have time to talk." "If I went to church, no one would notice I was there."

The depressed person does suffer from loneliness, but her problem is not the same as that of the person who is simply lonely. Neither is her problem the same as that of the grieving person.

Every person suffers significant losses during life, such as the death of a loved one, a business failure, or a loss of health. When we suffer such losses, we may have feelings of sorrow and distress. We call these feelings grief. Usually a grieving person will go through several stages. This process is normal. However, if a person gets bogged down too long in any one stage, her grief may turn to depression. At this point, the grieving person starts changing—maybe she'll quit eating or she'll start feeling hopeless about her future. She comes to a stop in life because of her grief.

Grief is similar to sadness. "Sadness is a normal emotion created by realistic perceptions that describe a negative event involving loss or disappointment in an undistorted way."[4] We all experience feelings of sadness and sorrow. To say we don't is to completely deny our feelings. When we experience sadness, there is usually a clear-cut reason we can identify. We lose our job, we feel rejected, a friend is seriously ill, or our child is having trouble in school. Whatever the reason, we can usually identify the source when sadness comes.

Depression is different. We can be depressed and not know the reason why.

Our perception may become unrealistic as the sadness of depression distorts things. For example, when a loved one dies, a valid reaction of grief or sadness would be, "I've lost him. I'll miss his companionship and the love we shared." This kind of reaction is tender, realistic, and desirable.

In contrast, a depressive reaction would be, "I'll never be happy again now that he has died. Without him, there is no life, no future." This kind of reaction causes a person to bog down in life.

Anxiety, loneliness, grief, and sadness are all emotions we experience. They can be good for us and enhance our life; or, if they become distorted and unrealistic, causing us to lose our desire to go on, they can turn into depression.

WHO GETS DEPRESSED

Depression is no respecter of persons. The rich suffer with it just as much as the poor. No age group or social class is exempt from it. No profession is exempt from it, although writers are notorious sufferers of it. (Now, they tell me!) Although depression may be related to thinking patterns, it has nothing to do with IQ. Considering the unpredictability of life, no one is immune from it.

Christians, too, get depressed. We are not immune from it, although we do seem reluctant to admit having it. I don't know why, since the Bible is certainly clear about the depressive symptoms of some great men of God.

Four Old Testament giants prayed to die, exhibiting a symptom of severe depression. Numbers 11 records Moses praying to God to kill him. Disgusted with the manna God was providing for them on their way to the Promised Land, the children of Israel longed for the delicacies of the Egypt they had left behind. They forgot the brick kilns, the task masters, and the sting of the whip. The accumulation of their complaints wearied and discouraged Moses, so he prayed to die. The burden he was carrying was too much for him.

Job, another one who prayed to die, was a man of loss. In the space of a single day, Job lost everything—possessions, servants, family. This was followed by grim, prolonged physical suffering that shook Job's faith to the depths. Job's suffering made him wish he had never been born; and he sought peace and release in death.

After Elijah's victorious stand against Baal, he fled from the wrath of Jezebel and requested to die (1 Kings 19:4). Jonah, too, despaired and wanted to die. Jonah was upset because God canceled his plans to destroy Nineveh; he wanted God to confine his love and mercy to Israel. It's interesting that both of these men wanted to die after a spiritual high point in their lives.

The Psalms, too, evidence a struggle with depression. The writer of Psalms 42 and 43 was a depressed person. He had been removed from the Temple of Jerusalem, a place where he went faithfully to worship God. Describing himself as "cast down," the psalmist confessed to God his feelings of despondency and asked for strength.

Clearly, anyone—including people of faith—can become depressed. There are, though, some people who seem to be more predisposed to having it than others. Not everyone succumbs to failures, frustrations, and losses with depression. Some manage to rise above these things with only temporary pain. But a certain proportion of people can't or don't. These individuals seem to have a built-in vulnerability for becoming depressed. Who are these people?

Some people seem to have an inherited tendency toward depression. Research in this area is incomplete, but is currently pointing toward the conclusion that a predisposition for depression may run in some families.

Or, predisposition toward depression could be due to a biochemical disturbance involving an imbalance of important substances in the brain.

Others seem to have a personality type that makes them

vulnerable to depression. This type reveals low ego strength linked with a rigid conscience development and a proclivity to guilt feelings. (That's me!)

Statistics give the impression that women may be more predisposed to depression than men. Of those forty million people who are depressed, two thirds of them are women. For every male diagnosed as having depression, there are generally two or more women. Some studies indicate as many as six females for every male. Whether the studies are done on people who seek professional help or on the general population, the statistics remain the same.

Women have come a long way in the last fifteen years. Our mental health level should be way up, and we should be feeling good about ourselves. But the truth is that depression today is clutching women as never before: 70 percent of the antidepressants are prescribed for women. More women are in therapy than ever before. There's been an increase in alcoholism among women. Women are also the major users of anti-anxiety drugs, such as Librium, Valium, and Miltown.

Some people tend to think of the depressed woman as the isolated housewife. The truth is there's no difference between depression rates of employed women and non-employed women. Both are equally prone to depression, and both get depressed over the same kinds of issues.

These statistics imply that women are hurting, and the broader implication is that women may be predisposed to having depression. A classic study in the field of depression concluded that women's lives may be at the root of women's higher depression rate. The way we feel, the way we think, the way we live—all this relates to our predisposition toward or against depression.

This implication must not be misinterpreted. A predisposition toward depression doesn't mean a person will have it. It simply means there is fertile soil present, just right for sprouting and growing depression. If a depressive seed is never planted in the fertile soil, then depression will not grow. The person could live her life and produce a fine garden and never know her soil might have been just right for growing depression.

Or, even if a depressive seed is planted, it may be swept away by another event much the same way a seed may be blown away by a strong wind. Or, the seed could sprout and then quickly die from lack of watering or lack of sunlight. Predisposition does not mean that having depression is a certainty.

A word of caution is needed. Depression is a weed, not a flower or a fruit—something that we would want to produce. Part of depression's subtlety is that it makes us want to treat it like a prize rose—nursing it and giving it our undivided attention, causing it to thrive. If given this kind of attention, it can choke out all the other beautiful plants and fruits in our lives. That's why we must increase our understanding of it. We must know its symptoms and its causes. We must know how to destroy it and to live free from it.

Because the way we feel and the way we live may have everything to do with our predisposition, we also need to understand ourselves better. We need to look at ourselves as the women we are.

If we understand ourselves and understand depression, we'll be able to live free of depression. What we understand, with God's help, we can control. When we understand, we lose our naiveté. We don't have to be victims, as I was, of an illness we know nothing about.

[1]Juliene Berk, *The Down Comforter* (New York: St. Martin's Press, Inc., 1980), p. 21. Copyright © 1980 by Juliene Berk.

[2]Frank B. Minirth and Paul D. Meier, *Happiness Is a Choice, A Manual on the Symptoms, Causes, and Cures of Depression*, p. 24. Copyright © 1978 by Baker Book House. Used by permission.

[3]Maggie Scarf, *Unfinished Business: Pressure Points in the Lives of Women*, p. 85. Copyright © 1980 by Maggie Scarf. Reprinted by permission of Doubleday & Company, Inc.

[4]David D. Burns, *Feeling Good: The New Mood Therapy*, p. 205. Copyright © 1980 by David D. Burns, M.D. By permission of William Morrow and Co., Inc., New York.

TWO

HOW TO RECOGNIZE DEPRESSION

If we are going to gain control over depression, we must be able to recognize the illness. If we are going to do battle with it, we must recognize the nature of the enemy. Depression is not an illness that can be detected by a rise in the thermometer. It often comes on gradually and unsuspectingly, so that a woman cannot look back and pinpoint the moment her depression began. Actually, it can gain a strong foothold before a woman may be aware she has it.

Depression is sometimes masked, hiding itself from the afflicted person and from others. In my first depression, I knew that something was wrong because I didn't want to get up in the morning. I'm a morning person—a "lark," not an "owl" by nature. To me the sweetest time of the day is the early morning, a time of quiet and freshness, a good time for studying, writing, and praying. When I no longer wanted to greet the day or even get out of bed, I knew something was wrong. I didn't identify the change in my behavior as depression because, as I've said, I didn't know anything about depression. Later, as the symptom began to fade, I used the word "depressed" to describe what happened, but I used it unknowingly.

A year later, I went to see a doctor for some lower back problems. I was also awakening very early in the morning and didn't have my usual amount of energy. Both of these problems, I attributed to my back pain. If I could get rid of the pain, everything would be all right. While waiting to see the doctor, I picked up a magazine and began reading. The magazine had an article in it about women and depression. Eagerly I read it.

I taught a women's Sunday school class, and I figured some of the members of the class might be helped by the article! I didn't connect the article with my present problems nor with my not wanting to get out of bed a year earlier. Along with the article was a questionnaire for women to use to see if they were depressed. I quickly scanned the list of questions, and, to my surprise, learned that I was depressed.

Depression takes on many forms. The appearances of the illness may vary from individual to individual, and reoccurring bouts of depression may vary with the same person. By the time my third depression came about, I was becoming more familiar with the symptoms. By now, after having it twice, I was reading about depression and collecting information. But the third depression was different from the other two. The third one was so different that my doctor had to make me see that I was depressed. If he hadn't, I don't know if I would have recognized it on my own. When I returned home from the doctor's office, I pulled the list of symptoms from my files. I had fourteen of the eighteen symptoms!

To learn to control depression in my life, I had to recognize the symptoms so that I could anticipate warnings of the illness. The symptoms are like red flags waving, DANGER AHEAD; they are indicators that something needs to be done.

Because a woman needs to understand depression to control it, because she can have depression and not know it, and because depression comes in different guises, it's important to know the symptoms. Contrary to what my experience indicates, they are clear-cut and recognizable. Wanting to recognize them makes all the difference!

Here are the major symptoms of depression. (A space has been left in front of each symptom for you to check if it is applicable to you. Some of us need an objective evaluation to convince ourselves we are depressed.)

_____ 1. *Feeling sad.* The general appearance of the depressed person is one of dejection, discouragement, and sadness. A depressed woman might describe herself as being blue, down in the dumps, or feeling that she just doesn't care about much anymore. Her facial expressions may take on a sad look—drooping mouth, downcast eyes, and wrinkled forehead. She looks tired, and her features are strained.

Passivity develops. The depressed woman loses energy. No matter what she does, she can't seem to feel anything but sad. She doesn't care if anything gets done. Dishes may pile up in the sink, beds may be left unmade, and dust may collect on the furniture. She may lose interest in her personal appearance.

I use the word "may" because some depressed women go right on looking nice and taking care of their homes. But they will carry their sadness in some way and be slowed down by it.

Every woman is bound to feel down in the dumps or sad at times, as we've already discussed in chapter 1. A woman may feel sad and not be depressed. But if her feelings of sadness persist for more than two weeks or if she develops some of the following symptoms along with sadness, then she may be depressed.

_____ 2. *Change in sleeping.* The most common *physical* symptom of depression is a marked change in sleeping patterns. It could be snapping awake in the middle of the night for no apparent reason. It could be awakening early in the morning and not being able to go back to sleep. It could be insomnia—not being able to fall asleep. It could be sleeping unusually often or too long. Even the quality of sleep that a depressed person gets is different. A depressed person awakens easily and responds to small noises that wouldn't disturb the nondepressed sleeper.

____ 3. *Abnormalities in appetite.* A change in eating habits is a symptom of depression. Usually the appetite decreases, and there is a weight loss. However, my appetite increased during my first two depressions. I kept thinking a couple of cookies and a cup of coffee would perk me up, and then I'd feel more like writing. The depressed woman may stuff herself compulsively, without experiencing increased appetite. The added weight will probably increase her depression.

____ 4. *Change in sexual desire.* The depressed woman may find sex less interesting and less pleasurable than she once did. Her capacity for orgasm may diminish. Her menstrual cycle may stop or be irregular.

The usual reaction for a woman who is depressed is to experience a diminished interest in sex during depression. There are some women, though, who experience a heightened interest in sex and become sexually indiscriminate. As in the case of the woman who increases her eating while depressed, this kind of behavior only complicates the depression, adding more problems.

____ 5. *Feelings of fatigue.* The depressed woman feels tired and rundown, without her usual energy. She frequently complains about feeling exhausted for no reason. She may feel tired and listless all the time.

Any woman is bound to feel tired, even for several days at a time, but she'll know *why* she is tired. The depressed woman feels tired, but doesn't know why.

____ 6. *Trouble concentrating and making decisions.* A person who is depressed loses her capacity for clear thinking. She may have trouble putting things into proper perspective; her thinking will be muddled. She may find it hard to read and hard to listen to others talk. She may have trouble making decisions; and no matter which ones she makes, they always seem wrong.

Some depressed people find making even simple decisions very painful, such as determining what clothes to wear in the morning or what cereal to feed the children. Once, in between services at church, I came upon a friend standing by the telephone. When I asked her what she was doing, Marilyn said, "I can't decide whether to stay for church or go home to be with Brett. He's home alone."

"Does your son want you to come home?" I asked.

"I don't really think it makes any difference to him," she answered.

"What do you want to do?"

She shrugged her shoulders and said, "I don't know."

I went on to the worship service and left her standing there trying to make a decision. She had told me sometime back that she was depressed. As I walked away from her, I wondered if Marilyn's depression was caused by her indecisiveness. Now, I know better. Her indecisiveness was a symptom, not a cause, of her depression.

It's extremely difficult for a depressed person to think clearly; everything in life seems blurred. Therefore, it is unwise to make major decisions during this time. One's lack of clear vision can lead to mistakes that would normally not be made.

____ 7. *Feelings of agitation or retardation.* Agitation is increased nervous activity such as pacing or hand-wringing or constantly moving about, unable to sit still. The agitated depressive is characterized by restlessness, pacing, and repetitive speech.

Retardation is motionless apathy. The depressed woman may feel unusually slowed down—as if it's too much trouble to move about. She may feel weighted down, as though she is dragging heavy weights with her everywhere she goes. "And why should I move about?" she thinks. "There's nothing much worth doing, anyway."

Retardation refers to a lessened ability to think, talk, move about, and even to recall recent events. She may speak in slow, halting sentences. Her facial expressions may be flat, fixed, and unchanging.

____ 8. *Feelings of irritability and resentment.* This symptom is probably the most understandable of them all. Who wouldn't be irritable if she felt weighted down all the time and couldn't get any sleep? She also feels more anger and resentment than is usual, and this contributes to her irritability. External pressures may seem overwhelming; she may feel consumed with responsibilities. She gets angry at the people who keep asking her to do things, but she's afraid to reveal her anger. She's afraid she might explode, clobber someone, or go to pieces. She's tied in knots over the struggle. Not being able to do anything about it, she turns her anger in on herself.

____ 9. *Feelings of discouragement and pessimism.* Pessimism or extreme discouragement in a normally positive person is a sign of depression. She may become petulant and distrustful or absorbed with topics of a melancholic nature. She'll take the gloomiest view possible of her situation; and when she does try to do something about it, any trifling annoyance will send her right back to her position of discouragement.

____ 10. *Self-deprecation.* A depressed woman is a woman of low self-esteem. She has a negative self-concept, expresses strong disapproval of herself, and looks upon herself as worthless. She has an exaggerated view of her own problems. "No one has ever felt like I've felt." "No one has suffered like I have suffered."

She suffers from guilt feelings because she is not living up to the expectations of others or herself. She takes on responsibility for acts and events which, realistically, are outside of her control, in an effort to fight her feelings of worthlessness.

The guilt she experiences is probably completely out of proportion to what she has or has not done. Guilt has its place in our lives, as we'll see in the next chapter; but the depressed person magnifies wrongs and feels guilty out of proportion to the act.

____ 11. *Feelings of inadequacy.* This symptom is similar to self-deprecation. The depressed person feels inadequate, and she's critical of herself. It's as though she suddenly realizes that she's much less attractive or less competent than she thought she was. She views herself as being deficient in qualities that are important to her, such as her appearance, intelligence, spiritual maturity, or her ability to manage her kids.

____ 12. *Brooding about unpleasant things that happened in the past.* "My heart breaks when I remember the past. . ." says the psalmist (42:4a, TEV). The depressed individual is very introspective. She's preoccupied with recurring morbid thoughts as she ruminates over the past. The same images keep jamming her head, coming back again and again. Her preoccupation is an excessive one in which she goes over and over all kinds of wrongs in the past, both real and imagined.

____ 13. *Crying more than usual.* "Day and night I cry, and tears are my only food. . ." (Psalm 42:3a, TEV). With depression comes an involuntary tendency to cry. A depressed woman may either cry often or feel like crying often. When I was trying to help a friend determine if she was depressed, I asked, "Are you crying more than usual?" "Sobbing would be more like it," Linda responded. For the woman who already cries easily, depression may mean what it did for my friend, an increase in intensity. For other women, it may mean crying for reasons that at other times wouldn't bother them.

____ 14. *Feeling needier than at other times.* The depressed woman feels desperately in need of help or reassurance from others. She feels deprived of emotional support. She craves affection and reassurance from others and may long for her husband or her friends to notice how miserable she is and come to her rescue. She feels rejected and unloved, completely out of proportion to reality.

The depressed woman may give the impression she doesn't need anyone. She withdraws from social activities. She stays near home. Actually, she does need others, but her low self-esteem and pessimism keep her from letting someone know how much she needs help. She's sure, if she makes an overture, she'll be rebuffed or laughed at or challenged.

In my case, especially during my first depression, I felt desperately in need of God's attention. I wanted him to send someone to my rescue. God knew I needed help, so why didn't he send someone?

Other Christians I've talked with felt an estrangement from God during their depressions, and yet, at the same time, felt a desperate need for his help. One woman said, "I desperately wanted Jesus to reach out in love and touch me." Some Christians doubted if they were ever saved, and even went so far as to make a second profession of faith in an attempt to bridge the awful feeling of separation. Other Christians wondered if the Holy Spirit were ever going to work in their lives again.

____ 15. *Suffering from physical complaints for which no medical explanation can be found.* The day I read the article on women's depression in the doctor's office, I was there for a new ailment. There was a medical reason for the lower back problems, in the sense that the pain could be traced to an injury twelve years earlier; but I had lived with it for those years without having to see a doctor. The sudden occurrence of the pain along with other symptoms was an indication of depression.

Gastrointestinal problems are frequent among the depressed. A woman may suffer from diarrhea, but more frequently she will suffer from constipation. She may suffer severe headaches, backaches, tightness in her head, rapid heartbeat, and heart palpitations.

These physical symptoms are what cause depression to come in different guises. One woman may have constipation, another muscle spasms, another severe headaches—and yet, all three may be suffering from depression.

Sometimes these physiological changes cause women to have an overconcern with physical illness. Many erroneously become convinced they have cancer or hypoglycemia. Actually, many of them would prefer to have a physical illness rather than admit to depression. I may be guilty of that. That day in the doctor's waiting room when I discovered I was depressed, my reaction was, "Well, I won't tell anybody." A physical illness is OK, we think, but an illness with emotional overtones is something to keep to one's self.

_____ 16. *Mouth feels dry or tastes unpleasant.* When a woman is depressed, she may find her mouth feels dry a good deal of the time. She'll continually want a soft drink or a cup of coffee or some kind of liquid to ward off the dry mouth. Or, she may have a persistent bad taste in her mouth. Either symptom is a sign of depression.

_____ 17. *Feelings of hopelessness.* Dr. David Burns says that hopelessness is as much a symptom of depression as a cough is a symptom of pneumonia. The depressed woman feels that nothing will ever go right again. She feels trapped by the circumstances that brought on her depression and can see no way out. In fact, says Dr. Burns, "The degree of hopelessness experienced by seriously depressed patients who have an excellent prognosis is usually greater than in terminal malignancy patients with a poor prognosis."[1]

Feelings of hopelessness do not mean the depressed woman's situation is hopeless. But with her inability to see clearly, along with her self-deprecation, she feels hopeless and can despair to the point of wanting to end her life.

_____ 18. *Suicidal thoughts.* For this symptom to be applicable, a woman doesn't actually have to have plans for suicide. If she does, her depression is a serious one. Her suicidal thoughts may begin with a heightened awareness of the absurdity of life. This kind of awareness makes her wonder if there's any point in going on. She may begin wishing she were dead. Her thoughts become preoccupied with death. She feels it would be better than putting up with her troubled self. Suicide looks, at times, like the only way to rid herself of her intolerable tensions.

A woman doesn't have to experience all eighteen of these symptoms to be depressed. If she has feelings of sadness (symptom #1) and three or more of the other symptoms, then she is depressed. From these symptoms, we can see that depression is an illness that affects the total person—physically, mentally, emotionally, and spiritually. The depressed woman isn't merely feeling sad, hopeless, inferior, and powerless—she is also experiencing a number of physiological and mental changes at the same time.

These symptoms may vary in their degree of severity. They may even be more severe at certain times of the day. Many depressives report a worsening of symptoms in the morning.

The degree of severity can range from a sad affect and painful thinking all the way to a complete loss of contact with reality (called a psychotic break). The more severe the depression, the more delusional the thinking. This occurs in order to compensate for the extreme pain of reality. We should not be frightened by the possibility of becoming psychotic. "Most clinical depressions do *not* reach the psychotic stage."[2]

UNIPOLAR VERSUS BIPOLAR DEPRESSION

To complete our understanding of what depression is and what its symptoms are, we need to make one more distinction. The depression we are discussing in this book needs to be distinguished from manic-depressive disturbance.

To make the distinction, picture in your mind a straight line. That line represents a person's average, normal mood. A significant drop below that line would be the depression we are talking about. It is a down time, a low mood. But suppose the mood rises high above the line and then swings far below, high again and below again. This up and down, from high to low, represents the manic-depressive disturbance.

Another way of making the distinction is in terms of "poles" of emotion. Manic-depressive disturbance is referred to as bipolar depression because its moods encompass two poles of emotional state, highs and lows. The depression we are talking about in this book is unipolar, referring only to one pole of emotional state, the lows.

The lows of the manic-depressive disturbance are very similar to unipolar depression. The person in the high part of the disturbance is driven, impulsive, hyperactive, and striving. He or she is expansive, friendly, with delusions of grandeur. The "high" person denies the existence of any realistic barriers to the realization of his or her dreams.

Both bipolar and unipolar disturbances are accompanied by periods of irritability; both may be accompanied by sleeplessness; and both make a person incapable of sustaining realistic contact with her or his environment.

Statistically speaking, unipolar depressions are far more common than bipolar depressions. Manic-depressive illness isn't pro-women, as unipolar depression is. Manic-depressive illness affects men and women in roughly equal numbers.

A biological predisposition for manic-depressive illness has been established. There is an inborn, inherited tendency toward such illness. Since this biological tendency was discovered, the drug Lithium has been found effective in treatment.

A biological predisposition for unipolar depression has not been proven. The causes of such depression are many, as we will see in the next chapter. Consequently, treatment is not a simple matter. Unipolar depression is understandable, though, and it can be controlled.

This is not to imply that unipolar depression is a simple

matter. On the contrary, it is complex. But if we can come to an understanding of its possessive nature, if we can recognize it when it moves in on us, if we can know what triggers it—then we will know how to fight it. For some, that may mean fighting to get over it. For others, it means fighting to stay free from it. Fighting depression means effort, lots of effort; but we have much to gain by it. For, in the process, we not only learn a lot about depression, but about ourselves as well.

[1]Burns, *op. cit.*, p. 344.
[2]Minirth and Meier, *op. cit.*, p. 27.

THREE
WHAT CAUSES DEPRESSION

My husband likes to illustrate a devotional talk of his with a cartoon he saw once in a magazine. The first frame of the cartoon shows a bridge with a sign on the side reading, "Load Limit: 8 Tons." The next frame shows a sand truck approaching the bridge. On the side of the truck is a sign showing the truck's weight, "8 Tons." The third frame shows the truck ready to start across the bridge and a blue bird flying down toward the truck in pursuit of a free ride. The final frame shows the blue bird landing on the truck as the truck crosses the bridge. When this happens, the bridge collapses. The bridge could support eight tons, but not eight tons and one blue bird!

This illustration can help us understand depression as a time of stoppage in life. If we think of ourselves as the bridge, depression is a time of emotional collapse when we no longer function as we once did. The truck represents what we are trying to support—our relationships, our commitments, our responsibilities, and all the stresses, strains, and joys that go with them. The question we want to answer now is: What are the blue birds? What causes our collapse? In other words, what causes depression?

LOSS

When it comes to women and depression, there is one word, more than any other, which names the cause. That word is *loss.* The depressed woman is someone who has experienced loss.

We attach ourselves to others—our husbands, our children, our friends—and when we lose the object of our attachment, we lose our moorings. We flounder, frantically treading water, terrified we are going to sink without our attachments. Our attachments seem to be what matter most. This is true of women who are full-time homemakers as well as the employed woman and the highly professional woman. "It is around attachment issues, more than any other sorts of issues, that depressive episodes in women tend to emerge."[1]

But what is lost doesn't have to be someone. The loss could be a symbolic loss, or the loss of a fantasy, or the loss of a concept. Perhaps a woman has based a large amount of her self-esteem on her looks, and as she begins to age, losing her youthful attractiveness, she becomes depressed over its loss. If the fantasy or concept was very important to a woman, or if her self-esteem was based on it, losing it can be very painful.

What is lost could include a loss of faith—a sense of being abandoned by God. "The disillusionments that come when virtue fails to be rewarded, when loved ones die and tragedies befall us in spite of earnest prayer, when the dark nights of the soul proclaim the absence of any God that cares, all bring an emptiness where formerly there was meaning. . . ."[2] My first depression resulted from this kind of loss.

My husband has considerable training in the field of higher education, including an earned doctorate. Bob was working as a registrar at a Christian university when he was fired the first time. Finding a new job was difficult, as the field of higher education is a saturated one. It's not unusual to have one hundred applications for one position.

We prayed and searched earnestly. After ten months, the only opening that came was with a nonaccredited Bible Training Center. Bob went to work there as the registrar and as a teacher. He taught preaching, teaching, and speech. Bob loved the job, but he was let go after one year with them. This time he was unable to get another position in higher education.

Through the years of studying and preparing for a career in higher education, Bob had a continuing love for preaching. We had met each other in seminary where Bob was studying, not for career preparation, but for his love for God's Word. With the doors to higher education firmly closed, Bob wondered if God was channeling his love for preaching into a full-time ministry. We talked with our pastor about it, and he, too, seemed to feel this was the case. Bob committed his life to the ministry, and we began earnestly to pray for a church position.

During the days of waiting that followed, I did not doubt that there would be a church for us. It would take time, but God would have one for us. But many of the letters we sent out went unanswered, and we received little help from people who knew us. We were viewed suspiciously. Anyone fired two times that close together must have something wrong with him! The Bible Training Center was of a different denominational persuasion than the church of which we were members. Our denominational churches were afraid to hire someone who had been employed there.

When Bob would get discouraged, I would remind him that God either had a purpose behind all this or he didn't. I clung to the belief that through all that had happened to us, God was weaving some kind of meaningful design. The way I saw it, that design meant preaching. Bob loved to preach, he had a seminary education, and he had taught preaching. His becoming a pastor made sense to me.

As the severance pay from the Bible Training Center ran out, Bob could wait no longer for a pastorate. He traded his temporary window factory job for a job as an executive recruiter. Executive recruiters find people for companies. They work on a commission basis; so, in a sense, the job is selling people. Bob aggressively went to work, and I "went to work" trying to figure out what had happened.

The world of selling people was a new experience for us after our years of being service-oriented through education and church. When Bob would come home from work describing the deceptive practices of some of the recruiters, or when he referred to himself as a "head hunter," I recoiled. Why would God put Bob in such a position? What was the good of all the years of education Bob had? While recruiting takes selling ability and is grueling work, it doesn't call for a doctoral degree.

When we added up three years of seminary, four years of graduate work, four different jobs in higher education, a call to the ministry, and an executive recruiter's job, it made no sense. Because it seemed to make no sense, my conclusion was that God had no purpose in it. Without the belief that he had a purpose for us, there was no reason to face the day anymore, and I became depressed for the first time. While my next two depressions would take on other forms and other issues, underlying them all was the loss of my belief that God had a purpose for our lives.

UNEXPRESSED ANGER

Depression for men and women thrives on feelings that are not expressed or acknowledged—feelings of anger, guilt, and grief. I want to examine unexpressed anger, guilt, and grief as they particularly apply to women.

Some women have difficulty admitting they get angry. Aggression and anger are considered unfeminine. Nice girls don't get mad. Christian women have the extra inhibition that Christians aren't supposed to get angry. Consequently, a woman may suppress all awareness of her own angry feelings because she shouldn't be the sort of person who gets angry. Inwardly, she may be in a state of fury, but she refuses to admit it to herself because anger is not going to be a part of her behavior.

On the other hand, she may know she is angry, but doesn't know what to do with it. We'll understand this more when we look at a woman's nature in the next chapter. Her nonaggressive nature and her desire to please people make it hard for her to express her anger. "I don't want to cause trouble," a woman thinks, so she bottles the anger within.

Feelings of anger, however, will seek some form of eruption—not necessarily volatile, but obvious. A woman with unexpressed anger may become irritable. "I feel like a keg of dynamite, ready to go off any minute." Or, she may displace the anger and get mad at herself, turning her anger inward. "I always do everything wrong. What kind of person am I that people can treat me this way and get by with it? Why can't I express my feelings?" All the fury turns inward. When it does, it may cause depression.

UNRESOLVED GUILT

True guilt is a valuable asset for living. It helps us when we hurt others or betray our own standards and values. God uses guilt to influence us to change our minds about what we are doing, leading us to repentance. If we never felt guilt, we would not follow difficult rules or standards, obey the law, or have good relationships with loved ones.

But if guilt is so valuable, why does it often lead to depression?

True guilt can lead to depression when it is unresolved, when we leave it alone and do not take action. Straightening out the wrong is sometimes all that is needed to cure our depression. How simple that sounds, and yet how difficult it is to do. Some of the most difficult words to say are, "I was wrong." How hard it is to accept ourselves as people, capable of doing some of the things we do!

Another way guilt may cause depression is to deny its

existence, to live as if it isn't there. Claire, a single woman, started seeing a married man from her office for lunch. They enjoyed each other's conversation. Their conversations eventually led to an affair. Claire told herself it was all right because they really loved each other. How could it be wrong when it felt so right? They were in love, and that was all that mattered. She understood his responsibility for his wife and children.

The man got transferred, and some months later, Claire became depressed. She told her doctor there wasn't any reason why she should be depressed. But there was; the guilt of the affair was taking its toll and appearing as depression. Guilt is going to have its effect in our lives, whether we recognize it as guilt or not.

There's another way guilt may cause depression. In this case, the cause is false guilt. False guilt is too much guilt. It is more guilt than is warranted by the circumstances; or persistent guilt out of proportion to the actual transgression; or guilt over something that is not our responsibility or under our control.

Dr. David Burns tells of a woman who had been experiencing false guilt for many years. She was a fifty-two-year-old elementary school teacher who was obsessed about two episodes of shoplifting that had occurred when she was fifteen.

> Although she had led a scrupulously honest life since that time, she could not shake the memory of those two incidents. Guilt-provoking thoughts constantly plagued her: "I'm a thief. I'm a liar. I'm no good. I'm a fake." The agony of her guilt was so enormous that every night she prayed that God would let her die in her sleep. Every morning when she woke up still alive, she was bitterly disappointed and told herself, "I'm such a bad person even God doesn't want me."[3]

Her exaggerated guilt over a kind of behavior that only happened twice in her life finally drove her to attempt suicide before seeking Dr. Burns' help. Dr. Burns says, "What she feels cannot be described as a healthy remorse or regret about the actual shoplifting, but an irresponsible degradation of her self-esteem that blinds her to living in the here and now, and is far out of proportion to any actual transgression."[4]

FAILURE TO MOURN

Loss is a part of life. No one escapes it. When loss occurs, it hurts. The natural emotional response to loss is grief. Grief is appropriate because grieving heals. This is indicated in the promise of Matthew 5:4: "Blessed are they that mourn: for they shall be comforted."

Grieving occurs with a death or with the loss of a relationship or with the loss of something very meaningful. Grieving is painful, but it is healthy. It prepares the way for believing in a new life beyond the loss. It creates a willingness to try again.

Grieving has stages including a middle and an end. If we bog down in one of the stages, our grieving can turn into depression. Or, if we refuse to grieve, we set ourselves up for depression.

Why would a person not want to grieve? There are several reasons. One reason is, to grieve means to acknowledge the loss. The loss may be one the person just cannot bear to admit or to accept. To grieve means, "I realize he [she/it] is gone."

A second reason a person may not grieve is because she is afraid of the painful feelings of grief. She may be afraid that, once she lets herself give in to grief, she may lose complete control of her emotions.

A third reason for avoiding the grieving process is mixed feelings associated with the loss. The daughter who neglected her mother in her later years might refuse to grieve. If she grieved, she would come face to face with her guilt. Or, a wife might want to avoid grieving because of the hostile feelings she had toward her husband. To grieve would be to acknowledge her anger, anger that she might not know how to handle.

A fourth reason is that our culture encourages us to be stoic, to hold in our feelings and show how strong we are. In our society, we feel compelled to be in control and to bear up bravely. We try to put our loss behind us intellectually and to redefine ourselves without working through our grief.

Christians particularly try hard not to grieve because we have associated grieving with *not* believing in the resurrection. We can't seem to grasp the concept that we can believe in the resurrection and still have difficulty adjusting to the *loss* of the person's presence here. If anything, working through our loss makes the promise of the resurrection all the more hopeful in our earthly lives. To not work through it is to set ourselves up for depression. We substitute the one for the other.

REJECTION

There is a tremendous love need in each of us. We want to be accepted and loved. When we are rejected, it is like being stamped "unlovable" or "unacceptable." To be repeatedly rejected or be rejected by someone who means a great deal to us can cause depression.

The rejection doesn't have to be real. As long as it is perceived as rejection, depression may result. When Bob tried to find a place in the ministry, we put ourselves in the position of being vulnerable. It's one thing to go looking for a job on the open market; it's another thing to go looking for a job among those you care about.

As soon as Bob committed himself to the ministry, our church voted to license him to preach and never followed through. The church never once asked him to preach. I had never been a member of a church that didn't ask a person to speak at least one time, once he announced his call. During the two years following Bob's commitment, our church had openings for three staff positions. According to the printed job descriptions, Bob was qualified for each one.

The third position was that of mission pastor. Early on in the planning for the church's mission, Bob was interviewed for the position. All we were told after that interview was, "We are not ready to hire a pastor at this time." Hope lingered with us. We lived in the area where the mission was being built, we had a heart for missions, and it would have been a good place for Bob to begin. Our friends and those in the church we worked with, for the most part, were aware of our interest in the mission pastorate.

About eighteen months later, the church made its selection. It was not Bob. When Bob didn't get the position, no one said a word to us—not the committee, not the pastor, not our friends, not those in the adult department we led. I did not get depressed over Bob's not getting the mission pastorate. What depressed me was the silence of those who knew us. Why didn't someone come to our defense? We had been members of that church for almost five years. Had no one seen any potential in us? Why didn't someone say, "I'm really sorry you didn't get the mission pastorate"? The subject was ignored as though Bob had not had an interest in the position. I interpreted the silence as rejection. We had been stamped "unacceptable."

Tim LaHaye says, "Many times the depression is out of proportion to the rejection, especially when the individual concentrates on the injustice of the rejection and his subsequent loneliness."[5] I'm sure I overreacted to our situation, but I tell this on myself for this reason: If the rejection hurts enough to the person experiencing it, no matter whether it is rational, it can cause depression.

FATIGUE

Depression doesn't have to be caused by something complicated. It can be caused by something as simple to understand as exhaustion. This was probably Elijah's problem when he prayed to die (1 Kings 19:4). After his stunning victory over the priests of Baal on Mt. Carmel and after fleeing for his life from Queen Jezebel, he was worn out physically and emotionally. In ministering to him, God started at the most basic level of need with food and rest, indicating that some of Elijah's problems were physical.

In addition to physical exhaustion, depression can also result from mental or emotional exhaustion. It can occur when we have had too much excitement, too much stimuli, too much tension, too much stress, or too many demands made on us. Depression is the body's way of reacting, "Hey, I've had enough. There's a limit to what I can handle. Give me time to unwind."

Depression can be caused by giving out more than we take in, when we exhaust our spiritual resources. If enough positive things that nurture and inspire us are not taken in, we overdraw on our spiritual resources. The result is spiritual bankruptcy and depression.

FEELING TRAPPED

While feeling trapped is not as frequent a cause as loss and unexpressed emotion, it does appear enough to warrant our talking about it. Feeling trapped means seeing no plausible way out of a dilemma. Feeling trapped means not liking any of the alternatives offered by our dilemma, or *not wanting* the alternatives. It's the sense of having no control over what has happened or is happening. It's the sense of being unable to remedy an intolerable situation. It can mean not wanting to make decisions.

Families headed by single women are among the poorest in the country; and their numbers, in light of increasing divorce rates, are growing. Factors contributing to their poverty are inadequate finances, lack of child support payments, and the inability of the women to earn income sufficient to make ends meet. Then, too, unless the women can afford child care, they may not be able to work at all. There is a high rate of depression among these women. Faced with raising children with little if any emotional and financial support, they feel trapped. They're lonely and weary of the unrelieved responsibility of child care and household maintenance and can see no way out of their situation.

UNREALISTIC EXPECTATIONS

Joyce Landorf, popular Christian speaker and author, says, "As we grow up, the *ideal* concept and the unvarnished *real* begin to clash, and when we begin to measure or compare the two, we are dismayed to find the *real* always wins."[6] Having our ideals shattered and seeing the harshness of reality can be devastating and can cause depression. Unrealistic ideals may have to do with our life, with our faith, with others, and even with ourselves.

Some of us have unrealistic expectations of life. Perhaps we thought that if we were good and honest, everything would always turn out right. Perhaps we thought that we would always be taken care of—somebody would always be there to care for us and to make the decisions.

Some of us have unrealistic expectations of what faith can do or what prayer can do and are disappointed when they don't work as we believed they would. Some of us have unrealistic expectations of the Christian life. For example, we think Christians should be happy all the time. Then when we do get upset, we feel as though we have failed as Christians.

Some of us are unrealistic in our expectations of others. A woman may have thought that the "right" man would meet all of her needs. She believed that once she met Mr. Right her life would be happy and blissful forever. It's unrealistic to expect one person to meet all the needs of another person.

Or, the depressed woman may have unrealistic expectations of herself. She is probably unduly hard on herself. When new responsibilities come along, like motherhood or the duties of a new job, depression may result from feeling unable to perform them adequately. She makes unrealistic demands on herself and doesn't allow herself to make any mistakes. When she does make mistakes, she tends to magnify them and exaggerate their importance. It's as if she looks at her faults through the end of binoculars that make them appear gigantic and grotesque.

LACK OF PURPOSE

Men and women need something to live for. That's one reason why being a Christian adds so much meaning to life. A Christian believes there's a purpose behind everything that happens to us. This makes all the details of our lives significant. When I stopped believing in that purpose, I floundered and became depressed. I had been a Christian for so long, I simply did not know how to live without a purpose.

We find ourselves floundering when whatever has given our lives significance disintegrates. It doesn't have to be something profound as long as it was part of the structure we depended on. Neither do we have to be conscious of the way that purpose held us. Sometimes, it was just there, as a part of our life, going unnoticed until it was gone.

Vera, whose marriage had ended tragically when she was pregnant with her third child, realized this loss when that third child left home at eighteen. Vera had done a marvelous job of raising her children. She had worked hard and developed a career. Her life was full with church and friends. And yet, she admitted to me when that third child left home, "I found myself feeling lonely and adrift for the first time in my life."

What Vera hadn't realized was that behind her activities of child-raising, career-building, and church-service was the purpose of "getting my children raised." When they left home, she looked upon her job as done—her purpose ended. Then came a time of floundering—a time of unwinding and taking a second look at life. Her next question was, "What do I live for now?" The answer came in time, but before it came, she experienced depression.

Loss, unexpressed anger, unresolved guilt, failure to mourn, rejection, fatigue, feeling trapped, unrealistic expectations, and lack of something to live for are the major causes of depression. There can be other causes. Whatever might be traumatic enough to shatter a person's inner self and make her not want to go on living can cause depression.

The causes of depression can be related to each other. Anger and loss often go hand in hand. Unrealistic expectations and fatigue are obviously related. But a separate look at each of the causes is necessary to understanding them. Understanding the causes can help us sort out the reasons behind our depression. As we do, two other factors need to be considered: timing and predisposition.

TIMING

What if the blue bird in the cartoon had landed on the truck several miles before it came to the bridge and then decided to fly away about the time the truck approached the bridge? Or, what if the blue bird had landed after the truck had crossed the bridge? In either case, the bridge would not have collapsed. The timing made the difference—although the weight of the truck, the landing of the blue bird, and the construction of the bridge all figured into the collapse. In other words, *when* these causes occur makes a difference as to whether they cause depression.

A woman may be completely resistant on one occasion, and then quite vulnerable on a subsequent one. She may be resistant to depression at the death of a loved one at some point in her life. Yet a death happening at another time may send her into prolonged depression. Sometimes the piling up of stresses with not enough time in between for us to fully recover makes us more vulnerable to the next trauma. The impact of a particular cause depends not only upon the force of the cause, but upon the person's own state of being at the time.

PREDISPOSITION

There is a point when any person would be overwhelmed by disaster. We all have our load limits. Painful experiences and emotional dilemmas appear in every person's life, but some seem to buckle under more easily than others. They appear to be predisposed to depression. Or, in terms of the cartoon, somewhere in the construction of the bridge there is a weakness. The question is, What caused the weakness? Were the materials used in the construction of the bridge weak? Was the bridge built wrong? Did the years of service weaken it? Were cracks never repaired correctly? We are not sure where the predisposition came from, but we do know it's there.

Predisposition to depression seems to run in families. Relatives of depressed individuals seem to have a significantly higher incidence of depression than do individuals in the general population. Continual research is being done to see if the cause is genetic or environmental.

> There is no solid scientific case that has been made which demonstrates that there is an inherited, predisposing vulnerability in recurring unipolar depressive illnesses. The evidence for a genetic basis for *any form of depression other than manic-depressive* disturbance has, so far, not been definitely established.[7]

Predisposition to depression may be caused by biochemical factors within the body. We know that biochemical disturbances are related to depression. We see this reflected in the physical changes that occur during a depression—changes in appetite, sexual desire, thirst, and sleep. What isn't known is whether the changes accompanying depression are caused by biochemical factors or whether the depression causes the biochemical disturbances.

Predisposition to depression may be related to the early environment of a person. Depression is tied up with feelings and self-image and one's life situation. Some mental health experts believe that subconscious, unresolved conflicts of childhood predispose a person toward depression.

Other experts say that a certain personality type is more vulnerable to depression. "Out of all the various personality types in our culture, there is one type that is more likely than any other to get depressed at some time in life. That type is the 'nice guy'—the person who is self-sacrificing, overly conscientious, overdutiful, hard-working, and frequently quite religious."[8]

Women, as we've already seen, tend to be more predisposed to depression than men are. This is not an implication of weakness; it simply means their reaction to the causes we've listed is more of an inward nature than a man's is. Research in the last few years into the natures of men and women shows that each sex predominates in certain types of illnesses. For example, men are more vulnerable to heart or blood vessel disease. Women are more vulnerable to depression. This doesn't mean a woman won't die of a heart attack or a man will not get depressed. What it does mean is that women appear to have a vulnerability to depression, so the chances of a woman's having depression are greater.

Why is a woman more vulnerable to depression? That is the question we want to answer in the next five chapters as we look at a woman's nature, the world in which she lives, the times in which she lives, her body, and her past. By looking at these things, we can better understand ourselves and why we are vulnerable. When we acknowledge our vulnerability and understand the causes of depression, we are prepared to defend ourselves so we won't collapse under our load limit.

[1]Scarf, *op. cit.*, p. 87.
[2]Roy W. Fairchild, *Finding Hope Again: A Pastor's Guide to Counseling Depressed Persons* (San Francisco: Harper & Row Publishers, Inc., 1980), p. 21.
[3]Burns, *op. cit.*, p. 180.
[4]*Ibid.*, pp. 180, 181.
[5]Tim LaHaye, *How to Win Over Depression* (Grand Rapids, Mich.: Zondervan Publishing House, 1974), p. 58.
[6]Joyce Landorf, *Changepoints* (Old Tappan, N.J.: Fleming H. Revell Co., 1981), p. 14.
[7]Scarf, *op. cit.*, p. 531.
[8]Minirth and Meier, *op. cit.*, p. 55.

FOUR
HOW A WOMAN'S NATURE AFFECTS DEPRESSION

Some mental health experts believe that a woman's nature underlies her vulnerability to depression. The way she is made and the way she feels have everything to do with her susceptibility.

In this chapter, we are going to look at those aspects of woman's nature which might contribute to her vulnerability. This chapter will *not* be a comprehensive study of woman's nature. It will cover only those aspects which might make a woman susceptible to depression.

Discussing a woman's nature is risky these days. To talk about her feminine makeup is to talk about her uniqueness. To talk about her uniqueness is to imply that a woman's nature is different than a man's. The talk of recent years is that there are no basic or inherent differences between the sexes, only socially imposed ones.

But the truth is that there are differences. In the creation account, God said he would make a "help meet" for Adam (see Genesis 2:18). "Meet" is an old English word meaning "suitable." God purposed to make a partner suitable for man. The literal meaning of the Hebrew for "meet" describes a helper "answering to" or "corresponding" to man. The implication is that man is incomplete without woman.

The two complement each other. Being complementary is different from being supplementary.

To supplement means merely to add to. No lack of deficiency is implied, nor is any idea given of a specific relationship between parts.

To complement means to make complete or make perfect. To complement is to provide something felt to be lacking or needed. The complementary natures of man and woman make the "one flesh" ideal of Genesis 2:24 possible.

Men and women are not alike in size, anatomy, or sexual function. Some scientists now believe that they are unlike in more fundamental ways. Men and women seem to experience the world differently, and it has nothing to do with the way they were raised.

The recognition of these differences does not imply that one sex is better or worse than the other. Recognition of differences does not imply inferiority. Neither does recognition of differences mean a person's destiny is predetermined. Differences do not imply type-casting, and *they should never be a basis for social inequality.*

Examining our differences can make us aware of our uniqueness. Understanding our uniqueness can help us live with ourselves. And, for those of us who are depression prone, knowing ourselves can make all the difference in learning to live free from depression.

As we look at our unique nature, we are looking at women *in general* and not one woman in particular. The aspects we are going to look at are drawn from studying women as a whole. We are not saying every woman is this way. The aspects appear more in women than they do in men; but in women, they come in varying degrees. In some women, they may not appear at all. If you think some of these characteristics do not apply to you, you may be right. They simply may not be a part of your individual nature.

On the other hand, don't be quick to dismiss these characteristics because they don't appeal to you or because you don't agree with them. Some of us may not want to identify with some of the traits listed here, but an objective look won't hurt any of us.

The differences in men and women have been narrowing over the years. Our social environment either brings our innate tendencies to full bloom or sometimes covers them up; so someday the picture may look different. For now, however, many women are struggling inwardly and being hurt. Their struggles and hurts have everything to do with their nature. It is for these women that this chapter is written.

WOMEN ARE SENSITIVE

The brain is divided into right and left hemispheres. The right hemisphere controls the left side of the body, and the left hemisphere controls the right. The hemispheres are responsible for the way we think.

The left hemisphere is the "verbal" brain. It governs language and reading skills. It processes information logically, step by step.

The right hemisphere is the center of our spatial abilities. It processes patterns of information instead of processing information step by step as the left hemisphere does. It links facts together to form a concept and links a series of concepts into a coherent whole.

Current research is beginning to suggest that there may be differences in the brains of men and women that are genetically determined. Researcher Jerre Levy says that studying the differences between male and female brains "is an exceptionally controversial area. For every experiment in the literature that finds differences, there's another one that doesn't, and vice versa."[1] Nevertheless, she and others in the field have found some interesting indications that men and women do not perceive the world in the same way. They feel it differently, hear it differently, and puzzle out its problems in different areas of their brains.

The following is a description of where the research seems to be leading.

Men are right-hemisphere oriented. That's why men have an advantage at visual-spatial tasks. Women are left-hemisphere oriented and consequently have an advantage at verbal skills.

Men and women also use their brains differently. "Men use their right hemisphere more efficiently than women do."[2]

The converse is *not* true. Women do not use their left hemispheres more efficiently than men. The male and female brains are not mirror images of each other. They represent two different ways of thinking and learning.

"The male brain is specialized. Men use the right hemisphere when dealing with spatial problems and use the left for verbal problems."[3]

"The female brain is not specialized."[4] The hemispheres of her brain work together on a problem. This working together gives a woman an advantage. She can work on a problem with both hemispheres, making her potentially more perceptive than men. A woman may talk in a corner with someone for ten minutes at a party. When she returns to her husband, she gives him a complete character analysis of the person. Her husband says, "But that's ridiculous! How can you know all about someone in ten minutes?" And the woman says: "I just know." Six months later she turns out to be exactly right.

A woman's perception may make her hearing superior to man's. She is sensitive to tones of voice and intensities of expression. She is extremely sensitive to the presence and variation of sound.

A woman can combine her perceptual and verbal abilities better than a man can, and she is good at reading faces. This makes her sensitive to a whole range of social cues and their meanings.

Females are sensitive to context, good at picking up information that is incidental to a task that's set before them. They are also able to absorb and later retrieve a good deal more peripheral information than a man can. They can pick up minute things that are not normally observed by a male.

Women are at an advantage in reading the emotional content of faces. Women can sense the difference between what people say and what they mean. They are good at picking up expressions that reveal another person's true feelings. Women can pick up unspoken thoughts, often understanding how another person feels. The perception of women is the result of both left and right hemispheres coming to bear on a single subject or person or statement.

WOMEN ARE PEOPLE-ORIENTED

From birth, females are more tuned in to other people than men are. Studies have shown that a female baby is more reactive and responsive to other human beings than a baby boy. Baby girls smile more. They are more responsive to the cries of other babies in the nursery. They start crying along with another baby more readily than baby boys do.

Baby girls babble more in response to the sight of a human face. At the age of three months, girl babies show great interest in and pay attention to photographs of human faces. Male babies, at the same age, can't quite distinguish between photos and simple line drawings of both normal and distorted faces. All stimuli are equally acceptable to male infants, while girls prefer photos of human faces. There's an innately stronger "other people" bias in even the smallest female.

While writing this book, I read an article about a woman chancellor at a major midwestern university. She makes $62,000 a year and maintains a working style that is totally executive. The article described her as one of the most powerfully and upwardly mobile women in the United States. In light of how the article praised her handling of the role, reviewing her many and demanding responsibilities, it was interesting to read how she evaluated her job: "I really like it when I walk outside and so many students speak to me. That's one of the things that pleases me. . . . Obviously, there are a lot of students I never see, but it is good to be recognized." Here is a highly successful woman who has made it in a traditionally male role, but who counts her success in terms of people. She's doing what comes naturally, because as a woman it's her nature to be people-oriented.

WOMEN FORM LOVE BONDS

A love bond, or attachment bond as it is sometimes called, is a force which unites people together—wife to husband, husband to wife, parent to child, etc. A love bond is characterized by strong and enduring affection. It's the holding fast and adhering necessary to achieve the "cleaving" or "one flesh" intended for husband and wife (see Genesis 2:24). It's the protective influence that a parent wants to have over a child. It's the cement that causes a friendship to endure.

Obviously, by definition, men and women both form love bonds; but they seem to mean much more to women than they to do men. Perhaps it's because a woman is people-oriented, or because of her ability to give singular attention to a relationship, that she places so much more of herself into a love bond than a man does.

In our culture, with its emphasis on individuality and independence, it is hard to comprehend the magnetic force of a love bond. A long-term perspective may make it easier to understand. Love bonds have been one of God's ways of preserving mankind. In earlier days, to live and to survive depended upon powerful social bonds. They kept otherwise vulnerable individuals in close proximity to protectors. Powerful attachments between the female and a mate upon whom she depended, between parents and their offspring, and between the family and the larger community were necessary for survival. Intense feelings for one another kept individuals near to each other. Their love bonds contributed to their survival.

Maybe we don't need love bonds as much anymore—or think we don't. But the instinct toward bonding is still with us. It goes right on operating in our lives, helping us develop relationships and enabling us to survive in this world. The bonds are so strong, we greatly resist any disruption of them. We do not give up our bonding without great psychological or physical anguish.

Women are powerfully invested in their relationships. They derive a sense of self from these vital emotional connections. Their inner selves become intertwined with others. Attachments matter to both nonworking and working women. The way they secretly view themselves and appraise their self-worth is in terms of relationships.

WOMEN ARE NOT AS AGGRESSIVE AS MEN

Men seem to have an inborn masculine "aggression factor." Some would put it this way: men are always ready to fight. Contest is the pattern of life for them. It is instinctual; they appear to be hormonally primed for aggression.

In light of this aggression factor, Cecil Osborne calls man a "do-er." Man has a need to conquer and achieve. He is an activist—an experimenter, an explorer, a builder, a competitor. (Part of this drive to "do" is also related to the contribution of his brain's right hemisphere.)

Although there are individual women who equal or surpass men in ability to do many of these things, women generally lack the *drive* to do them. A woman finds her fulfillment more in what Osborne calls "be-ing." She does not always have to be doing something or always proving herself. She can conquer, but she finds it much easier being herself. This sense of being gives her many lovely qualities. It makes her warm and sympathetic—something that someone who is always competing finds difficult to be. It makes her a peacemaker. In accord with her sensitive nature, it enables her to feel an unusual oneness with nature, with people, and with events.

To say that women do not have a drive toward aggression is not to say that women do not have aggressive feelings. Far from it! Women experience aggressive feelings, and they can be aggressive when necessary; but there is an innate aggression factor within men that women as a whole do not possess.

In the harsh, competitive society in which we live and work, we certainly need the qualities of sensitivity, caring for people, enduring relationships, and nonaggression. Our world needs the influence of the unique attributes of women. These qualities can make such a positive contribution to life, that it is hard to believe they can also contribute to depression. But they can. Here's how.

DEPRESSION AND THE AGGRESSION FACTOR

Through the struggles with Bob's career—first the firings and later the unsuccessful attempt to enter the ministry—Bob never got depressed, but I did. The reason for that can be explained by the differences in our natures.

Bob's desire to provide for his family *drove* him and kept him going. He always had something to do, something to conquer. When he was fired the second time, he immediately went to work at a window factory to supplement the severance pay. Simultaneously, he was looking for positions and planning ahead for the church he would pastor. There were days of extreme discouragement, of anxiety, and of depressive *feelings;* but never did Bob reach the point of clinical depression as I did. When he became an executive recruiter, a job paid in commissions, the drive he had to provide for his family spurred him on. He did not have time to stop and consider God's purpose in the same way I did.

The days Bob worked at the window factory were heavily

invested days for me emotionally. I wrote Bob's letters for him, encouraged him at night, and was caught up in his dreams about the church in our future. When he decided to go to work as an executive recruiter, the decision was made on a Friday and he went to work on Monday. Bob took all the energy of his confusion and plowed it into his new job. The energy previously used for job hunting was now used for earning a living. I was left holding a heart full of emotion that I didn't know what to do with. What was I going to do with the emotional energy I had invested? Not realizing what was happening, I turned inward with the emotional energy. The result was depression.

Both men and women experience aggressive feelings, but they don't handle them the same way. Because men are hormonally primed to conquer and to do, they tackle the setbacks in life in a similar way. When men fail, their nature is to fight, to challenge, to endure. When women experience setbacks or failure, they respond emotionally or become depressed. Women may feel powerless to do anything and react by withdrawal and silence. Underneath they may be seething, but they can find no acceptable outlet for their feelings.

For those who see themselves as powerless, depression can even be a way of power in itself. Sometimes, a person will see that when she is depressed, people pay attention to her—friends, husband, family members, etc. In seeing their reaction, she subconsciously begins to see depression as a tool for power. Depression becomes a tool for fighting a battle that a person feels she cannot otherwise fight. In some cases, her suffering is all she possesses to gain some control over those around her or perhaps punish them for their lack of love. Attention in a negative way, she feels, is better than no attention at all!

Some people, both men and women, learn to fake depression early in life. Then when they need to, they put themselves into a temporary depression in order to manipulate people. They do this when they want attention or to punish an authority figure for not letting them have their own way.

When it comes to the aggression factor, depression can result when a person doesn't know what to do with aggressive feelings and when it can be power for the powerless.

DEPRESSION AND THE PEOPLE FACTOR

I never suffered depression over the rejection of Bob from two jobs when he was fired. I never suffered depression over the rejection he received from the churches he wrote to. But I did get depressed over the rejection he experienced at our own church. I cared about what the people in our church thought because I cared for them. We could be stamped "unacceptable" by people I wasn't close to or didn't have a personal relationship with, but I couldn't handle it around those we knew well. I know now that I based too much of my self-worth on what my fellow church members thought of me. Because women are people-oriented, it is tempting for us to base our self-esteem on what others think.

To be people-oriented is to be tempted to translate success in terms of what others think. Good feelings about ourselves become dependent upon the esteem of those around us. A woman's feelings of well-being, her sense of worth, are hostage to the attitudes and approval of others or perhaps one very important person.

Depending upon what other people think is dangerous. People can change their minds. One day they want one thing, another day it may be something else. Constantly to depend on and evaluate oneself in terms of what others think makes a woman in danger of losing her identity and therefore very vulnerable to depression.

DEPRESSION AND THE LOVE BOND FACTOR

You may have noticed in this book that when I said Bob was turned down by our church for three positions, I said,

"We were rejected." When I said Bob was fired, I said, "We failed." That's the nature of love bonding for a woman. She so intertwines herself with the one or ones she loves that what they experience, she experiences. What hurts them hurts her. Their agony becomes her personal agony. If anyone would have told me before marriage and parenthood how deeply I could feel, I would never have believed it. Through the commitment of marriage and the raising of children, God has stirred such deep feelings within me—so deep that I didn't know it was possible to hurt so intensely.

A woman puts so much of herself into her relationships. She cements herself to the ones she loves. And very often, without even realizing it, her very identity gets wrapped up in her love bonds. Who she is has meaning in terms of whom she loves.

Depression for women, when it occurs, happens in one kind of context more than any other. This context is the loss of the love bond or relationship.

> It is around *losses of love* that the clouds of despair tend to converge, hover, and darken. Important figures leaving or dying; the inability to establish another meaningful bond with a peer-partner; being forced, by a natural transition in life, to relinquish an important love-tie; a marriage that is ruptured, threatening to rupture, or simply growing progressively distant; the splintering of a love affair or recognition that it is souring and will come to nothing. . . .[5]

A woman's love bonds are her joy, but they are also her sorrow. Rupture and disintegration are not exceptions any more, they are cultural norms. For every three marriages entered into, more than one ends in divorce. Our children grow up to leave home. High mobility rates spell loss of extended family ties, friendships, and stable supports. Women generally outlive men by seven years, some say eight years. Losses and disruptions are a part of living. You would think we would get used to it, but we don't.

We resist with great biological force any disruption of our attachments. We do not give them up without great anguish. Sometimes our relationships or one such relationship constitutes everything in our world. The loss or threatened loss of that attachment can be experienced as a devastation of our own self. We're afraid that if the relationship ceases, there won't be any way of *being* any longer. The loss of the attachment feels like death itself because our entire being has been defined in terms of attachment. The attachments are such a part of us, and so powerfully experienced, that we often respond to their loss or disruption with depression.

DEPRESSION AND THE SENSITIVITY FACTOR

Look again at some of the phrases describing a woman's perception—"zero in on a problem with both hemispheres," "more perceptive about people," "sensitive to tones of voice and intensities of expression," "good at reading faces," "absorb and later retrieve a good deal more peripheral information," "sensitive to context," "good at picking up incidental information." In many areas of life, these traits really come in handy. We can be sensitive to our husband's needs, to our children's, and to our friends'. We can be sensitive on the job in meeting the needs of customers, in knowing how to please the boss, and in running an efficient organization.

But, honestly, there are times when I wish my sensitivity didn't work so well. I wish I could be unobservant for awhile. My sensitivity may be another reason why I became depressed over our church's rejection, while Bob did not. I read the silences. I took in what was not done for Bob as well as what was. I collected hurts to add to our hurt. I saw things that Bob did not see although we were both there together, observing the same things.

While I don't believe a woman's sensitivity is actually a cause of depression, like the loss of a love bond or unexpressed aggressive feelings, it can be a contributing factor. When the cause for depression is already there, it can deepen the cause and make it worse. In some cases, it can possibly even distort the cause, making it more unjust than what it actually is.

Being sensitive, being people-oriented, investing ourselves in love bonds, and being nonaggressive are some important parts of our uniqueness as women. They add much to the richness of our lives. At the same time, they can make us vulnerable to depression. The way we are and the way we feel has much to do with our high depression rate.

[1]Jo Durden-Smith, "Male and Female—Why?" *Quest*, October 1980:15-19, 93-98.

[2]Joyce Brothers, *What Every Woman Should Know About Men* (New York: Simon and Schuster, 1981), p. 39. Copyright © 1981, Joyce B. Enterprises, Inc.

[3]*Ibid.*

[4]*Ibid.*, p. 40.

[5]Scarf, *op. cit.*, pp. 86, 87.

FIVE
HOW A WOMAN'S WORLD AFFECTS DEPRESSION

The aspects of woman's nature we just considered—sensitivity, people-orientation, love bonding, and nonaggressive drive—are things which twentieth-century science is telling us about the innate differences of men and women. Sufficient studies have been done to support each aspect.

Now let's look at some aspects that aren't as well supported—aspects that would be hard to prove. These aspects are the conclusions of psychologists and counselors who have worked with men and women and observed them over a long period of time. In considering these aspects, our purpose is not to try to prove them or even to convince anyone of their rightness. Rather, our purpose is to shed more light on the vulnerability of women to depression.

These aspects are more environmentally oriented than those we considered in the last chapter. They have everything to do with how women were raised and with the world they now find themselves in. As our world changes, these aspects may change also; but for now they have a lot to do with the unhappiness of women.

A lot of articulate people speak out on how it should be for women; but many women are still struggling with "how it was" and "how it is." "How it was" is that women have been seen as nurturers; as learning many "shoulds"; as having low self-esteem; as taking things personally; and as desiring security.

1. *Women are nurturers.* In the past women have been viewed as nurturers. This is understandable in light of their finely tuned emotional skills, their interest in people, their intense love bonding, and their ability to give singular attention to something.

We more often think of nurturing as specifically relating to child raising. Certainly, this has been true in the past. But all women do not have children. Some women do not marry. Some who do marry do not wish to have children. That equipment for nurturing, however, is still there, seeking to surface in some manner.

Their nurturing quality keeps women from being deterred from the demands of a particular goal. A woman can nourish and support a goal, bringing something beautiful or meaningful out of overwhelming odds. A career woman stays with a difficult project and pulls the snags out of it, astonishing her fellow workers. A woman takes over the most difficult Sunday school class in the church, fourth through sixth grade boys, when everyone else has given up on them. In a few weeks, she has the boys eager to come to Sunday school and happily learning. A woman who has grown children has a hobby of raising house plants. She exclaims, "I've just got to have something growing—something to care for." To bring something along, to care for something, to train, to support—these skills come naturally for most women. They are nurturers.

2. *Women learn many "shoulds."* "Shoulds," such as "You should tell the truth," and "You should obey your parents," are beamed at both boys and girls. But by the time those boys and girls are adults, the message gets twisted until women have often been pushed into seeing themselves accountable for everything. No one knows for sure why this is.

The reason could be simply that girls learn the "shoulds" better. This may be because of their sensitivity, their verbal skills, and their ability to sit still. Boys, with their drive for aggression, just may not be able to learn enough self-restraint to respond as well to the "shoulds."

On the other hand, it could be that boys in the past were given more latitude. Not as much was expected of them as was expected of girls. "Boys will be boys," was the attitude.

A third possible explanation is that maybe parents wanted to protect girls more and so more restraints were put on them. Whatever the reason, the result is adult women feeling responsible for everything. (Remember that personality type prone to depression? She's the one who is overly conscientious, overdutiful, and hard working.)

I've often said that my conscience works overtime. I know so many "shoulds" that, at times, I've looked upon them as a curse. In high school, one of my favorite teachers taught me this saying: "There is but one failure and that is not to be true to the very best one knows." That saying describes my effort in life, always to do everything the best way I know how.

A very noble goal. And yet the longer I have lived and the more responsibilities I have assumed, the more difficult it has become to do my best. It is impossible to be the "best" in all my roles—wife, mother, Sunday school teacher, speaker, writer, gardener, housekeeper, friend, daughter, etc. I know a lot about "how" each one is to be done, but I cannot live up to my knowledge. That's frustrating, because guilt wants to ride along, hounding us for all those things not done to our utmost. Living up to the "shoulds" in our lives, or experiencing guilt over not living up to them, can be a heavy burden to shoulder.

3. *Women are of low self-esteem.* There is a way of viewing events called the "attributional style" that is common to depression-prone people. Healthy people blame a failure or disappointment on external things—like bad

luck—and they figure it's a temporary state. People who become habitually depressed blame themselves and believe that this personal shortcoming will affect everything they try to do.

Women in general appear to have this depressive attributional style more than men. In a social psychology experiment involving a puzzle that couldn't be solved, women students said they couldn't solve it because they were stupid. But male students said they didn't have enough time or it wasn't fair.

A similar response is often made in the loss of a love bond. A woman will frequently blame herself. No matter what happened, she is often readier to experience guilt, anger, and reproach against herself than blame the other person. If she is disappointed, then the real cause lies in her own unacceptability, inferiority, unworthiness, unlovableness, and guilt.

Christian women are not immune to low self-esteem. Joyce Landorf was asked by *Christian Life* magazine what she thought was the greatest problem of Christian women today. Her answer was that it is the problem of low self-esteem. Landorf first identified this problem over ten years ago when she began speaking frequently to Christian women. She says that, since that time, she has seen lots of people speaking out about the problem and trying to deal with it, but she has not seen much improvement.

Low self-esteem isn't an altogether bad starting point. The Bible shows us how God used people of low self-esteem to do great and mighty things (Judges 6:15, 16; 1 Samuel 9:21; Exodus 3:11; 4:1, 10; Luke 1:48). Low self-esteem can be a channel for God to work through, in which we depend upon his strength to do a job. Low self-esteem may initially prepare us for living the Christian life; but we must be cautious. Too much low self-esteem, in which we have no regard for ourselves and in which everything becomes our fault, can be unhealthy and lead to depression.

4. *Women tend to take things personally.* Closely related

to the problem of low self-esteem is the trait of taking things personally. Here's the way "taking things personally" works:

You have a friend who is a real estate agent. The two of you talk on the phone several times a week, usually at her initiative, since her schedule is more varied than yours. Suddenly, she doesn't call as much. You try to call her. No answer. You think, "What did I do wrong to cause this break in our relationship?" (The truth is, business had an upswing for the real estate firm, and she was simply busy.)

You and your neighbor often get together for coffee at ten-thirty. You both have toddlers, and the coffee break gives you a time to visit while your children play. One day as you start to leave the house at the usual time, you see your neighbor and child pulling out of the driveway. You think, "She must be tired of my coming over. She could at least have told me." (The truth is the neighbor's toddler fell just a few minutes earlier and cut himself. The neighbor is taking the child to the emergency room. She didn't have time to call to let you know.)

You have an old friend in an influential position who has agreed to help you find a job. In one week you had to call him three times about job matters. The last time you call is on a Friday afternoon. As the conversation ends, he says, "Now don't call me this weekend." You tell your husband, "Some friend he turned out to be. He was just pretending to want to help me." (The truth is the friend was going out of town for a very important business meeting. If you had called him that weekend, he would not have been home.)

Women who take things personally find it hard to look at themselves and what happens to them objectively. They find it hard to laugh at themselves. They have a one-dimensional look at life in which everything that happens is directly related to self. A three-dimensional view is healthier, in which we can see the interplay of events involving others besides ourselves.

5. *Women usually desire security.* Every person desires

some security, but women seem to want it more than men. Cecil Osborne says, "The need for security is one of the strongest emotional needs a woman possesses."[1] By security, Osborne doesn't mean simply financial security, although for some women that may be part of it. Osborne says a woman wants to be taken care of, protected, and provided for. She wants her relationships and her world to be stable and satisfying. She wants the stability provided by a close family unit—husband, children, home, and enough money to maintain the operation.

A woman may make terrible bargains in life in order to be taken care of. She'll tolerate enormous amounts of unhappiness and misery to avoid losing what she *perceives* as her security.

A friend of mind stayed with a marriage long after there was any hope of salvaging it. For over twenty years her husband cheated on her; he was a gambler and an alcoholic. Marion did everything she could to make the marriage survive. She was the picture of the submissive wife as described in Ephesians 5:22, 24. Any woman is going to fear for her future in the event of the breakup of her marriage; but Marion's fear seemed excessive.

I couldn't understand her excessive fear since she was an attractive, capable woman. I failed to see how life without her husband was going to be any worse than life with him. From my vantage point, she had already managed a lot of her life without him; yet Marion was wracked with fear that she would never get a job. She was petrified she would never make it on her own.

In trying to encourage her, I'd say, "Marion, you'll love the woman you're going to be."

After her divorce, she found a good job and was able to manage her home extremely well. She made a good adjustment, found single friends, and took good care of her children, even riding out some rough problems with them. Everything about her spelled CAPABLE WOMAN.

Two years after her divorce, I said to Marion, "Now, aren't

you proud of the woman you've turned out to be?"

"Yes, I am," she slowly answered. "Actually, I realize now I was handling more than I thought. I wasn't as dependent as I thought I was."

There was a long pause. Then Marion continued, "But I still worry about the future. I still want someone to take care of me."

PRESSURES OF THE WORLD THAT IS

When we looked at some aspects of a woman's nature in the last chapter, we were saying, "Here's the way a woman is." In this chapter, we have seen a woman as she *may* be. Now our question is, "Can she be the woman she wants to be in the world in which we now live?" Can a woman be herself?

We live in a world (speaking of the United States) in which individualism is of prime importance. We live in a world where manly qualities such as aggression and conquest are revered. We live in a world where success is sought desperately. These pressures exert themselves on women. They say "Here's the way you should be."

Today's world says, "You ought to be making money." Money has become a criterion for evaluating a woman's work. It's not a matter of comparing salaries, trying to determine who is making the most money. Rather, it's a question of, "Do you get paid for what you do?" The impression is, if you do anything of any importance you are going to be earning money.

A backlash of this pressure is a putdown of motherhood. Mother's job no longer has status in a society which rewards the single-minded pursuit of money and success. The role of mother clashes head-on with the real values of an achievement-oriented culture. The implication is, "You're wasting your time if you are not earning money." The world is saying, "Deny your nurturing self unless there are monetary benefits."

In response to the pressure to make money and the desire to nurture and to have close personal relationships, a woman may try to combine the roles of mother and employee. She can do it, but it won't come without cost. There will be tension as she juggles the demands of the two, for there are harsh conflicts between the demands of a career and raising a family, no matter how fulfilling and rewarding both may be. Both demand time, energy, and resources. Children need more than spare-time mothering; and bosses don't want to pay full-time wages to part-time workers.

All of a woman's "shoulds" rise up within her, flashing on and off, reminding her that she should be a good mother. They also remind her that she should be a good worker. But there's not enough time and not enough energy for the woman to be as good at both as she knows she "should" be.

As we think about working for money and employment, we need to make a distinction between the two kinds of working women. There are those women who have a "job," and there are those who have a "career." Those with a job often don't have to put so much of themselves into it. The job is simply a task to be done as one does other things she is responsible for and wants to do. There's a difference between this kind of working and the hard-nosed, aggressive activity demanded for pursuing a career in the business world.

Being her hard-working self is enough for the first kind—those with simply a job. But much more is required for career building. A woman must also learn corporate politics, competitiveness, and assertiveness. If she's going to get anywhere, she's going to have to fight for it. Some women may get weary of the fight.

While working on this book, I read a newspaper article about women who were leaving white-collar managerial positions for blue collar jobs. In management, they didn't like the continual struggle between people. They simply wanted to go to work, do their job, and go home. Their actions are understandable in light of what Osborne said about women whose nature it is "to be." They are peacemakers, wanting oneness with the people they relate to.

This same world that is beeping the messages, "Make money," and, "Be employed," is also saying, "Be an individual." The message says to do your own thing; your happiness is what matters most. The world that beeps this message laughs at dependency. Independence and individuality are what count. A woman's nurturing nature and her tendency to put people first are directly opposed to individualism. To have meaningful love bonds and meaningful nurturing experiences requires some dependency. A woman affected by this pressure may want to be close and affectionate with her family and friends, but is afraid she will be too dependent on them. She wants one thing, but feels like she has to act another way.

Whoever started beeping the message of individuality to women was probably trying to do them a favor. Women who viewed themselves as "doormats" for their children and husbands needed some individuality! They needed to know they had rights, and that it was all right to assert those rights. Somewhere, though, the message became distorted into a message that emphasizes self. A woman who is largely people-oriented is not going to find happiness when she becomes the center of her own attention.

Putting self first is also contradictory to Christian values. Jesus said that greatness in the kingdom of God would be determined by putting others first (Mark 9:33-37). Individualism pressures Christian women because it contradicts their nature and their values as Christians.

Both the employed woman and the at-home woman usually feel the pressure to keep a clean house. A woman has a lot to be responsible for. She often assumes the greater responsibility for relationships, for the activities of the children, for cooking, cleaning, church activities, paying the bills, etc. Many of the things she does seem to lead nowhere.

The clothes she washed will get dirty again. The dishes she wipes will be used again at the next meal. The dust will come back. The floor will have to be vacuumed again—the jobs are endless.

While much is being printed on fathers becoming equal caretakers of the home, the truth is they usually are not. We occasionally get a report in the media about a man here or there who is doing his share; but the majority are not. This is not a putdown of men. Often they simply do not see a lot of things that need to be done. Remember that eye for details women have that we talked about in the last chapter? There are a lot of details to caring for a house—details that men don't intentionally overlook. They just don't see them or remember them.

And some men, those who are earnestly pursuing a career or who are in business for themselves, don't really have time to look after all the details. If the wife also chooses a demanding career, the tension can spark over who is going to take care of the essentials of living. This is not to say that there aren't solutions; but they don't come about without struggle.

As if being pressed to keep a clean house, be an individual, and be gainfully employed aren't enough—the world is also saying, "Be beautiful." I can remember when we looked upon the pressure to be attractive as a worldly influence. Gratefully, we acknowledged, God looks on the heart. We knew God was more concerned with inward qualities and our service to him than he was with how we looked on the outside.

Now, according to some, God looks on the outward appearance, too. The emphasis is, "If we really want to please God, we're going to be slim, have an up-to-date hairstyle, learn how to apply makeup skillfully, and wear the right colors. Our devotion to God can be gauged by our appearance."

I was reading one of my husband's books written by a Christian man talking about the needs and struggles of men as they approach mid-life. One chapter was written to women. The author talked of some of her pressures, like those I've just mentioned. The author's solutions for the needs and struggles of men were varied and sympathetic. For women, his solution was for her to just work on her appearance, exercise, and improve her looks; then her problems would be solved. When I read that I threw the book across the room!

I do understand a woman's desire to be as attractive as she can be. What I'm questioning is the implication that her attractiveness measures her dedication to God or that improving her attractiveness is *the* solution to her problems.

One more pressure (and there are many) I would like to mention may be unique to Christian women. That's the pressure of having a good marriage and raising balanced children. Somehow, the New Testament message of submissiveness has been twisted to give the impression that, whatever has gone wrong in a married woman's life, it was because she wasn't submissive enough. This impression isn't entirely the work of male, authoritative preachers. A lot of material written for Christian women by Christian women gives the impression that a woman can have a perfect family and a perfect life—if she'll submit herself to her husband's authority in all things.

One woman, struggling to raise some step-children who were being very difficult, was told by her Sunday school teacher that the reason she was struggling was because she wasn't being a submissive wife. Where was the responsibility of the children's mother for the years she had had them? What about the father's responsibility? What about the personalities of the children?

Submissiveness is a beautiful principle that enables men and women, two very diverse creatures, to live in harmony. Someone has to have the final authority in the home or there will be chaos; but being submissive is not a panacea for all of a wife's problems.

I've been working with women in small groups for a long

time. I've seen enough heartache in women's lives to know that submission doesn't solve all problems. Life for women is just too complex for us to believe and teach that all of their problems can be solved with the application of this one biblical principle.

With all these pressures being exerted on a woman—to make money, be employed, be an individual, keep a clean house, be beautiful, have a happy family—no wonder her inner cry becomes, "What about me? Isn't anybody ever going to accept me as I am? When is it ever going to be all right to be the woman I am?"

RESULTING DEPRESSION

After looking at how a woman is, how she might be, and how she should be, let's see if we can make a connection with the causes of depression.

Loss—relationships, which mean everything to a woman, are constantly changing.

Unexpressed anger—anger at being asked to do too much; anger at always having to do for others without someone caring in return; anger at being taken for granted.

Unresolved guilt—A gal I really admire surprised me by saying, "I love my job. I believe I'm where God wants me to be. I wouldn't want it any other way; but there's always the guilt."

"Guilt? Guilt over what? You are the last person I would expect to have a problem with guilt."

"Guilt over leaving my kids when they were small," she answered. "I stayed home with each of them a year, and then I just had to get back to teaching."

Failure to mourn—failure to express grief over the loss of a relationship.

Rejection—in trying so hard to please others, she's programming the message back to herself, "I'm unworthy. I don't measure up."

Fatigue—One newspaper columnist in reviewing a book

that alleges superwomen will one day take over the world said we didn't have anything to worry about. "Most of today's superwomen are just too tired to change the world."

Feeling trapped—the woman who feels guilty over leaving her children, but can't quit because the family is dependent on her earnings. Or, the woman who intensely dislikes her job, but is afraid to face the insecurity of looking for another one.

Unrealistic expectations—all the "shoulds" blink on and off and a woman keeps expecting herself to be the "best" in all situations.

Lack of purpose—her desire to please others begins to look like manipulation to her. Everybody around her controls her with their demands so that she doesn't know who she is or what her role is any longer.

We may never be able to prove that a woman's nature and her world underlie her vulnerability to depression; but we will have to admit—they provide fertile ground for it.

[1]Cecil Osborne, *The Art of Understanding Your Mate* (Grand Rapids, Mich.: Zondervan Publishing House, 1970), p. 50.

SIX

HOW THE TIMES IN A WOMAN'S LIFE AFFECT DEPRESSION

The depressed psalmist talked of his soul as being "cast down" (Psalm 42:5, 6, 11). "Cast down" is a shepherd's term. Phillip Keller says it refers to a sheep that turns over on his back and cannot get up again. The sheep finds some little hollow or depression in the ground and lies down in it for comfort. The sheep is fine if he just lies there; but if he rolls on his side slightly to stretch out or relax, the center of gravity in his body shifts and his feet no longer touch the ground. In this position, it is quite impossible for the sheep to get up again. The once active, healthy sheep is immobilized because of his choice to lie down in what he sees as a comfortable stopping place.

Part of the shepherd's work is to rescue the "cast down" sheep. How much easier his work would be if his sheep grazed on a terrain where there would be no little hollows or depressions in the ground to tempt them. But terrains aren't that way. Even the smoothest of pastures have tempting, grassy spots just right for curling up.

The terrain of life for a woman has just such "curling-up" places—places where she wants to stop for a while.

Her curling-up places aren't places of rest. They are places of contemplation about where she is in life and about herself. Often she enters a place filled with reluctance and fear. She is reluctant to part with an old way of life and afraid to move on to another. If a woman lolls too long in her curling-up place, it may become a "cast down" place for her. Her contemplation may become depression, and she'll need help in getting out just as the cast-down sheep does.

The shepherd cannot predict where a sheep will be cast down; but we can make some predictions about where our cast-down places may be. Depression can appear at any time in a person's life; however, if we look at women as a *group*, we'll see many in the same age span being depressed about similar issues. Their depressions reflect the underlying issues and concerns of a particular time of life.

As we go through the different age spans, noting the cast-down places, we are not charting the lives of women. Most lives do not follow a straight line which can be broken down into stages. The lives of women are full of sudden discontinuities and surprises. There is usually far more shifting of direction in the life of a woman than in that of a man. The life of a woman is rarely neat and predictable.

Perhaps, in an earlier time, when every woman's life more or less followed the same pattern, it could have been charted. Today's woman has choices—lots of them. Having choices hasn't necessarily made life easier for her. Her choices have complicated her life, and, at times, even brought her to cast-down places. The choices have to do with: "Who am I?" and "What do I do?" Then later, her agony may be over: "What should I have done?"

By looking carefully at the hollows and crevices that are potential cast-down places, we can see where we are and perhaps gain some insight into pulling ourselves out. We can also be better prepared for handling the cast-down places ahead of us, as we gain an understanding of the nature of a woman's life.

THE ADOLESCENT WOMAN

The first cast-down place a woman meets comes during adolescence. On first glance at individual cases of adolescent depression, they look similar to adult cases: rejecting relationships, school problems, a move, loss of a family member, or too much stress. A deeper look behind adolescent depression reveals that it revolves around two things: (1) detachment from parental authority; and (2) achievement of an independent self that's not emotionally merged with the parents. In other words, adolescence is the process of separating self from parents.

Adolescence is when a woman is going to encounter serious loss for the first time—loss of childhood and of her childhood self. Letting go of her first love bond, her dependency on her parents, and of the child part of herself is distressing. The realization of the finality of the end of childhood creates a sense of urgency, fear, and panic.

If you are the mother of a teenage daughter or the friend of a teenager, you may be thinking, "Well, I never noticed her having such feelings." That may be true, because the adolescent is not talking about these feelings. She's absolutely certain no one has ever felt this way before. We can catch a glimpse of these feelings in what one young Christian woman wrote in some unguarded moments. She wrote these words in the spring of the year, a month before she was to graduate from high school.

> It arrived so quickly; yet it took forever. I have been waiting impatiently for the last twelve years. I thought it would never come. And then—suddenly—it's only a month away. It comes like spring. All winter you long for spring, and then—without warning—it's here. Your heart aches from trying to cram and hold so many wonderful memories in your heart. You don't want to forget because any day now it will be summer. You want to remember each smell, each blossom, each walk, and each new blade of grass. You know you can't, and it makes your heart hurt.

> In a month, I will be graduating. I'm frightened! I want it to all be over and yet, I want to hold on to each little thought. I'm miserable because I don't want tomorrow to come. The more I see of adult life—the more I want to grow younger. Tagged to each thing I do is the thought, "It will never be like this again."
>
> I know how the little sparrow must feel when he first tries to fly. He's terribly frightened and would rather stay in the nest, but there's something within him saying, "I want to fly. I want to soar high above everybody."
>
> I, too, want to fly. I want to do things—new things. I'm frightened—yet, impatient. I have one thing, though, in which I can be confident. As surely as the Heavenly Father watches over the little sparrow, I know he is watching over me. With this, I face the future.

The "it" she refers to in the first line is not graduation. "It" is the moment of separation—of leaving self and a way of life behind and moving on to being a new, independent self. Her ambivalent feelings are obvious. She is reluctant to give up the past; but, at the same time, she wants to. She is afraid of the future and yet excited about its possibilities.

The ambivalent feelings are quite normal. For good mental health, it is essential that this separation take place and that the adolescent becomes her own person. Mourning is a natural part of this process.

> Mourning is, in and of itself, a wound-healing process of a psychological nature. That is to say, grieving involves a time of mental hurting and agony which has its wonderful human resolution: true mourning ends with what is called internalization, a "taking in" of the person who has been lost to us. It is thus true that, in the fantastically complicated process that goes on during adolescent separation, we are *parting psychologically* from our parents—with pain and with suffering—but in doing so, *making them a part of ourselves.*[1]

The process of separation affects both males and females, but it seems to take a far greater toll on females. Three times as many adolescent girls as boys *attempt* suicide. Unrealistic expectations and pressures of today's world contribute to the adolescent woman's despair. She is caught between the traditional stay-at-home mother role and the new frontier of freedom. Consequently, she's pressured toward fulfilling all the possibilities the changing world has to offer. As one teenage girl said, "It used to be OK for girls to sit back and let things happen. But now you have to be competitive, pretty, smart, go to college, be an executive, and still have men find you attractive."

Fear will cause some adolescents to try to remain indefinitely in this period of development, making it a cast-down place. The teenager becomes depressed because she is afraid she won't be able to survive the rupture of the love bond. She becomes depressed because she's afraid she won't be able to make it on her own. The hazardous condition of this cast-down place is not to be taken lightly because, if unresolved, it can be a trap for future depressions in a woman's life.

THE WOMAN IN HER TWENTIES

If adolescence could be summarized as a period of mourning and fear, the twenties could be summarized as a period of choices. The choices revolve around selecting a mate, what kind of commitment to make to him, and whether to have children.

If a young woman's adolescence was complete and healthy, she then searches for another love bond after separating from her first one with her parents. Finding a mate is often a major concern of the woman in her twenties. Her new identity will be dependent upon this bond.

> It is only *after* a woman has achieved security and a sense of worthfulness in her love relations . . . that she is released

> from her "unendingly anxious" feelings about her personal value. It is only when she's achieved security in an ongoing emotional attachment that she becomes truly internally liberated. . . .[2]

Establishing a love bond with someone of the opposite sex doesn't mean the woman in her twenties is engaged in a frantic search for a man. On the contrary, she is engaged in many endeavors and enjoying them; but ever riding in her thoughts is the possibility of marriage—when and with whom. Her self-worth sometimes hangs in the balance as she waits for this issue to be resolved.

When a woman's love bond with a mate is established, her next choice is what kind of commitment she is going to make to him. Is she going to use her energy and abilities to help her husband meet his goals? Or is she going to use that same energy and those same abilities to pursue her own goals?

That "singular attention" a woman can give to something or to someone is hard to divide. It is a hard decision to give that singularity to her husband and neglect her career. But since bonding is so important to her, as is wanting to please her husband, it is hard *not* to give him her singular attention.

She may choose to give her attention to her husband, supporting him and what he wants. Or, she may try to be supportive of him and pursue her own goals at the same time. This will be like trying to develop two selves. It can be done, but it won't be without struggle and tension.

Sometimes the struggle becomes too much, and the young woman simply gives in to one or the other. She may choose to give up her career and commit herself to her mate. Or she may choose to give up her mate. As one recently divorced professional golfer said, "When I was on the golf course, I was constantly thinking about him. When I was with my husband, I was constantly thinking, I ought to be practicing my swing."

This choice of commitment is not resolved with a one-line oath at a certain point in time in which she swears allegiance to her career or to her husband. This choice is more like an internal war involving conflicting feelings. The war may involve many inner battles until the young woman is able to discern the kind of commitment she wants to make.

A third choice for the woman in her twenties is whether to have children. We are living in the first period of human history in which women are able to control to some degree their reproductive life. Unplanned and unwanted pregnancies have been largely avoidable since the development of the birth-control pill.

Gone are the days when a woman has a child as a matter of course soon after she marries. Today, women consider carefully their own lives—their careers, their emotional readiness, their finances before considering parenthood. Women go through harsh soul-searching over whether to be pregnant now, later, or never: "Should I have children? When should I have them? How many? If I choose career over motherhood and children, will I regret it? How does my husband really feel about children?"

If you've already made the choices of the twenties, you may tend to downplay the agony you went through deciding about a mate, commitments, and pregnancies. (How could the choices of the twenties really have been cast-down places?)

I responded that way, too, until I started really thinking about my twenties. I remembered the hours spent praying and wondering over God's will. While there was never a question for me as to what kind of commitment to make to my mate, I did spend an awful lot of time praying about marriage (if, who, and when) and about how many children to have.

My choice about how many children to have came at a time when the campaign to "stop at two" was in full force. I can see now that my contemplation over this had the potential for becoming a cast-down place. There was anger in me. If I had been born twenty-five years earlier, I could have had all the children I wanted. There was guilt. The implication was that if you are a responsible, caring person, you won't have more than two children. There was loss, because I erroneously equated stopping at two with turning off motherhood. See the potential for depression?

The dilemma of choices is frustrating for the young Christian woman today. She wants so much to do the right thing. External forces are saying, "Here's the way you should be." Internal forces may be challenging that with, "But here's the way I am." She must then ask herself over and over, "What am I going to do in light of the opposing forces?" If she can't resolve the question, she may find herself in a cast-down place.

THE WOMAN IN HER THIRTIES

The thirties can be characterized as the years of the turnarounds. After making the difficult choices of the twenties, a woman in her thirties now wonders if her choices were the right ones. No matter which lane she chose to travel down life's highway—the traditional lane of commitment to marriage and motherhood or the lane of commitment to a career—her thirties find her questioning her choice. It is as if she looks over to the other lane, and suddenly decides she's driving in the wrong one.

The woman who chose to stay home, who saw herself as a loving, nurturing mother, now wonders what she might have missed by not working. As her children enter school, she finds herself not being needed as she once was. She looks now at the working world as a place of fulfillment. If she has set aside goals in choosing to stay home, those goals surface again at this time, beckoning her to make a change.

The woman who chose the nontraditional lane is experiencing a similar struggle. She looks at the full-time homemaker and wonders if she missed something. Maybe the glamour of commuting to the office every day has worn off. Maybe she's tired of the rat race and being responsible for her share of the bills. Maybe the freedom she wanted so much now feels confining.

Maybe she put off that choice about having children. In her thirties, she sees time to have a family running out. The passing of age thirty signals to a woman that her prime time for reproduction physically has passed. The statistics for her own well-being and that of her baby are starting to go against her. She realizes she cannot continue to procrastinate in her decision about having children.

As the middle thirties approach, she knows deep down there are very few women who want marriage who don't now have it. There are very few women who want children who don't now have them. She now has to come to grips with the fact that many of her options are no longer available. The adolescent years and the early twenties were wrapped with a golden glow—she always had choices. In the thirties comes the startling realization that one's options are closing. This realization may be very hard for a woman to deal with. She may grieve over not having exercised certain options. She must now make a meaningful adjustment to a life with closed-off options.

The underlying theme of the turnarounds of the woman in her thirties is the crashing of the assumptions on which she had been living her life. She assumed she was making the right choices. She assumed she could always have children. She assumed she would always be young. That these are false assumptions becomes consciously real during the thirties.

Whether we acknowledge it or not, we all have assumptions on which we base our actions. We might never have articulated them or even thought about them, but they are there just the same. Our assumptions are challenged in our thirties as life becomes more demanding and unpredictable. Our commitments demand more of us than we ever thought possible. Hopes are seriously diminished. We begin to see that our dreams aren't going to come true.

Many of the assumptions Bob and I had about the Christian life came crashing down through his employment at the Christian university and the Bible training center, through our membership in a large, success-oriented church, and through our many efforts to enter the ministry. One of our assumptions was that if we followed God in every venture of life, then all would go well with us. This didn't mean we would always understand what was happening to us, but it did mean we would always have the regard and respect of our fellow Christians. We attempted to be sincere, conscientious Christians. We worked hard, did our jobs quietly without fanfare, had a simple life style, and were family oriented.

One of the first things we were told in trying to find a church was that it will depend on who you know. Well, we didn't know anybody! In our attempt to be conscientious Christians, we had not given thought to trying to make "connections" for our future.

We were further surprised to learn how untouchable we were as failures. The implication is, if you are really a person of faith, everything will go well for you. If it doesn't, then something is wrong with you.

Churches wanted leaders who could guarantee success. Stepping into the ministry was stepping into new territory; the likelihood of failure was always present. We could not guarantee success. All we had to give a church was our love, our sincere desire to serve the Lord, and our ability to teach God's Word. Those qualities, we learned, were not good enough.

In the way of a reaction, I became critical of many of the religious leaders who were deemed successful. It did not seem to matter what kind of life some of these leaders lived. The "sheep" seem to make no distinction over what kind of "shepherd" they would follow. If the leader's words were spoken with authority, if they were preceded with,

"God told me. . . ," then they were accepted and followed whether or not the words were in accord with the nature and teachings of Jesus. Power and personality in the leader were the important things. It looked as though what it took to succeed in the Christian realm was the same as what it took to succeed anywhere—assertiveness, successful image, political connections, being a good promoter and a people-manipulator.

I brooded over how naive I had been to have believed it could have been otherwise. Being conscientious and having a sincere desire to serve the Lord were not enough to keep a job in a Christian setting or to enter the ministry. With the loss of my naiveté, I also lost my sense of wonder. In their places came cynicism and depression.

Don't underestimate what the *loss* of one's assumptions about life can do. In this age group we see the highest depression rate for women. Today's typical depressed woman is in her thirties, white, educated, and married. Her world may appear solid to those who know her, and yet the assumptions she lives by are disintegrating, and she finds herself in a cast-down place.

THE WOMAN OF THE MIDDLE YEARS

The difference between the cast-down places of the thirties and of the middle years is the difference between assumptions and roles. Assumptions have to do with our perceptions of life. For example, we perceived ourselves as always having options. Roles have to do with our ways of being. The cast-down places of the middle years are role related. They have to do with the loss of our roles and with our roles changing. Let's look at four potential role-related cast-down places of the middle-aged woman.

1. One potential cast-down place is the loss of the mother role. Not every woman, not even every woman who stayed home to rear her children, experiences depression as the nest empties. The concept of the depressed woman with

the empty nest is a grossly overstated one. One sociologist interviewed one hundred and sixty women and found that all except one responded to the departure of their children without any problems. It was the husbands who suffered more when the children left home! The men had had little time for the children when they were growing up and sometimes had not had much interest in them. When the children left, the fathers were full of regret.[3]

Some women, though, are overly affected by the departure of their children. Who are these women? They are women who interpreted their meaning as a person in terms of being a mother; women who have remorse over the kind of mother they were; and women who refuse to mourn over the loss of their mother role.

If a woman saw herself as being important only because she was a mother, or if all of her energies were directed toward being a good mother, that panic of "Who am I going to be when the children leave home?" will make her vulnerable to depression.

Likewise, the woman who has remorse over the kind of mother she was will also be vulnerable. Perhaps she kept thinking, "Tomorrow there will be time to do things with the kids." Tomorrow never came; and in her middle years, she realizes that it's too late.

The woman who refuses to acknowledge the emptiness sets herself up for depression. She prides herself on being stoic or on being so professional that motherly things no longer interest her. In other words, the natural thing is to experience some grief over the loss. To do the unnatural is to set herself up for depression.

2. Another potential cast-down place of the middle years is the loss of physical attractiveness. Some women become depressed over the aging process and the loss of youthful looks. In a sense, it is like the loss of a relationship. The woman pines for the youthful, sexually appealing person that she used to be. She is filled with a sense of emptiness and grief as though abandoned by her lover.

A woman like this has probably used her attractiveness to obtain interest in herself and to receive positive feedback. She is probably limited in her capacity to relate to other people, because in the years previous she depended upon her looks to gain attention and establish contact with people, especially men. With the loss of her looks, she also loses her feminine power to attract.

This may be why the fortyish single woman is much less satisfied than the single woman in her twenties. Culturally, our society says older men are distinguished and interesting. Older women are just old. Socially, she is no longer in demand as the "extra woman"; while the single man who is fortyish has become a much more sought after item.

3. Another potential cast-down place is the loss of the person you might have been. This is the stage of life in which a woman reviews what she has actually done, compared with her original hopes and plans. As Ellen Goodman puts it, "At twenty, I wanted to know who I would become. By forty, willy-nilly, ready or not, I've become."

As a woman reviews the past, she may conclude that her life hasn't really amounted to much in comparison with the starry-eyed expectations of youth. She may resent abandoning the past. As she moves in a descending direction, she estimates what have been her profits and what have been her losses. As she looks toward a shrinking future, she estimates what hopes, if any, might still be realized.

Giving up the past along with its dreams and facing a shrinking future can be exquisitely painful. Along with this, she must come to grips with her own mortality. Her life on this earth will not last forever. If a woman cannot successfully resolve this crisis of feelings, she may experience intense bitterness and disappointment so profound that it may lead to depression.

4. Another area of vulnerability to depression in the middle years is an increase in role responsibilities. The middle years could be described as the years of "too much responsibility." Middle-age has bosses to please and deadlines

to meet and bills to pay. Middle-age has both aging parents and adolescent children or children who may be beginning their own families. The problems of children these ages are more heart rendering than the problems of children in younger years. The problems have far more serious consequences coming at a time when parents must exert a different kind of influence on them. A woman, who is usually the flexible one in the family, is always changing to meet all of these needs. She may feel she's unable to hear enough, be enough, and do enough for those she cares about.

Loss of role and loss of power coming at a time of increased responsibility make the middle years of a woman's life full of potential cast-down places.

THE WOMAN OF THE LATER YEARS

The utmost depressive item of women beyond age sixty which must be faced is potential widowhood. Men on the average die seven to eight years earlier than women. If a woman has not cultivated any way of living apart from the marriage bond, widowhood can be an extremely troubling time. Most women, however, will have developed a strong sense of self by the time they lose a mate through death. This does not mean the loss of a mate will not be agonizing. It will, and these women will grieve over this loss, but with a strong sense of self. They will not despair to the point of not wanting to go on with life. They will work through the grief and learn to live peaceably alone.

Retirement, for a woman, isn't the major depressive issue that it is for a man. A woman does not derive as much of her identity from a job as a man does. By the time she reaches this age, a woman has many ways of being. She finds fulfillment in various ways and so is not overly dependent upon a job for her identity. Her diversity makes her retirement years more fulfilling than most men's. (Of course, this fulfillment may be marred by a husband who is depressed because *he* has retired!)

The depression rate is low in the later years. By this time, a woman has usually worked through the issues that make for depression. Her later years are ones of inner harmony. If she hasn't worked through these issues, she may despair in grieving over "what might have been." Indeed, she may find herself struggling over accepting the finality of this life. She may feel time is too short for the attempt to start another life and to try out alternate roads. She may not have had the life she'd wanted. Now, in her later years, she comes to the depressive realization that she will not have another.

Looking at the cast-down places in a woman's life helps us understand ourselves and helps us see when we may be more vulnerable to depression. Some of us need this look to help us understand why we are now depressed. The cast-down places help us see our reluctance to give up one way of life and move on to another. Others of us need this look to prepare for the future. Our reaction is better when we step in a hole we know is there than when we step in a hole unsuspectingly. If we know it is there, we watch our step to see that we don't get hurt. If we don't know it is there, we may break a leg. Understanding makes all the difference in how we handle our potential cast-down places.

[1]Scarf, *op. cit.*, p. 29.
[2]*Ibid.*, p. 225.
[3]Brothers, *op. cit.*, p. 251.

SEVEN
HOW A WOMAN'S PAST AFFECTS DEPRESSION

A woman's nature, her world, and the times in which she lives make her vulnerable to depression. Looking at those items is like examining the foliage of a plant to determine what it needs to grow. Not all the causes of difficulty are on the surface—there are others, not readily distinguishable. If no obvious cause for the plant's condition can be gleaned from its color, its leaves, or its stem, and if it is getting plenty of light and water, we assume the problem resides below the surface. Perhaps the roots have rotted or the soil needs fertilizer. Something is going on underneath the soil, causing the lack of proper growth.

Likewise with depression, a woman's vulnerability may run very deep. "A person who becomes clinically depressed for the first time at age forty in all likelihood had some contributing roots to his depression planted at age four."[1] This is true for men and for women; but in this chapter, we are going to look at the importance of the past from a woman's point of view.

UNCARING PARENTS

We have already seen how depression is linked with self-worth and low self-esteem. It is an illness of self-deprecation. Where do we get our self-esteem? Where and when does a person gain a healthy sense of self-worth?

The sense of one's worthfulness—of being an all right person who has value and who matters greatly to another—comes, initially, from the loving relations a child experiences in the family. In other words, a child's self-esteem derives from having been cared for by his or her parents. Not to be loved is, for the young child, much the same as to be no good.

> Parents who are overly strict can also cause low self-concepts to be developed in their children. The child assumes the parents are correct and he blames himself for not being perfect. . . .
>
> A child with a cold, rejecting mother and a passive or absent father will also have a low self-concept and be prone to depression.[2]

The motives behind the strictness of the parents may have been noble, but it is how they registered on the screen of the child's brain that causes the damage. "Whether the child's perspective is real or imagined, once he suspects that his parents do not approve of him or, worse yet, wish they had never given birth to him, he becomes a likely subject for depression. . . ."[3]

LACK OF A MOTHER'S LOVE

A mother's presence is necessary for *psychological* survival of human babies. "Babies who are regularly fed and well-housed, but *are unable to form a bond with a caretaking person*, show astonishing and alarming mental and physical deficits."[4]

The early love bond with our mother forms the foundation of our personality. Babies show a strong drive to form an intense emotional connection with a caretaking figure.

> This need to create a bond or tie with mother first manifests itself at about six or seven months of age. The love-bond that comes into being somewhere around this period becomes even stronger and more absorbing and exciting: it reaches its peak of intensity, for the child, during the second year of life. What is called "attachment behavior" (that is, behavior directed toward keeping the parent close by) becomes slightly less exaggerated after about the age of three; but it is still very much a part of the scene until the fourth or fifth year. Thus, from infancy onward and to about the fifth year, much that the child *does* is . . . directed toward a single and overriding goal. And this is keeping the caretaking and guardian mother as closely at hand as is possible. The baby experiences her presence as "satisfying" and "security-enhancing."[5]

The mother who exudes love unconditionally, who gives her child, despite all the turmoil and irritation of the day, the full-bodied and reliable mother-warmth that child craves, has provided her with a basis of feeling she will carry throughout life. If mother-love is thwarted by circumstances or lack of enthusiasm, a child can be emotionally maimed for life.

LACK OF FATHER'S AFFIRMATION

In working with women as a Sunday school teacher and a prayer group leader, I noticed that many women who had integrated personalities and who handled the stress and strain of their environment well were women who had a good relationship with their father. Each woman had received her father's approval as a person in her formative years. This observation was confirmed by mental health experts when I researched depression.

> In some subtle sense this act of winning the parent of the opposite sex seems to be an important factor in helping

> the small child to achieve a sense of maleness in the little boy, or femaleness in the girl. When a girl fails to "win" her father, either because he is not affectionate or because he rejects her, or for some other reason, she often grows into a woman who has doubts about her femininity. Her femaleness has not been "ratified" when she was young. Something is missing in the feeling tones of such women.[6]

A girl receives confirmation of her desirability as a female and affirmation of her value as a person from her father. The way he treats her communicates to her his pleasure in her femininity.

As a girl's consciousness of self develops, she needs her father's continual affirmation that she is a worthwhile person. If she is denied his companionship, if she is denied the esteem and grace he can give her, this will be reflected later in her adult years. This lack of father approval has its devastating effect on our subconscious. It is hidden there and reveals itself later in different ways—ways that are related to depression.

Lack of a father's approval may reveal itself as a distrust or hostility toward men. Repressed anger or hostility, we learned, is an open door to depression.

Lack of a father's approval may reveal itself as a lack of confidence in herself as a woman. Low self-esteem is another door to depression.

Searching for that approval she missed may cause a woman to find herself in one hurtful situation after another. There's always a question mark in her mind about her worth. One woman in one of my classes was always finding herself being hurt. After several talks with her, I asked her, "What kind of relationship do you have with your father? In all the times we've talked, you have never once mentioned him."

A fierce look came across her face. Very tersely, she said, "We didn't have any kind of relationship." And then, to add emphasis, she clenched her fist and shook it in the air. "Just once, just once," she added, "I'd like to know I have his approval."

She was a mature woman and a fine Christian, but the hurt planted by her father's rejection many years earlier was still present in her subconscious, taking its toll.

DEALING WITH DEEP DEPRESSIVE ROOTS

In looking at the roots of vulnerability to depression through uncaring parents, lack of a mother's love and a father's approval, we have seen the almost limitless power parents have to lower or raise their offspring's self-esteem. In light of this, some cautionary things need to be said.

To react depressively to uncaring parents, to a lack of mother's love, or to a lack of father's affirmation is not necessarily inevitable or universal. Many children have lived under such circumstances and have endured with a strong sense of self. If you are depressed, don't readily make the diagnosis that you were unloved as a child or that your father ignored you. These kinds of causes may be fertile soil for deep-rooted vulnerability to depression; but they are not to be diagnosed by amateurs.

Likewise, don't use this information to make you feel worse about yourself. This kind of explanation is not to encourage you to look back and say, "Oh, how could my parents have treated *me* that way? How could my father have ignored *me?*" In most cases, what was done was never intentional. If you find the times in your life distressing, isn't it possible that your parents did, too? What you interpreted with your childlike mind as rejection may have been nothing more than your parents being totally wrapped up in their own problems.

Neither should this information make you think that you cannot get over depression and stay free from it. Looking back and blaming your parents should not be a cop-out for your depression. Your attitude should not be, "Well, my mother didn't love me," or, "My father ignored me so I can't help but be depressed." We are looking at our past to *understand* our vulnerability, not to give ourselves an excuse for our behavior or to point a finger of blame.

LOSS OF A PARENT

If a mother's love and a father's affirmation are sorely needed for good mental health, then the absence of one of those parents is definitely going to have its repercussions. The loss of a parent in childhood may lead to an increased vulnerability to depression in adult life. By loss, of course, we are speaking of the death of a parent. The loss, however, could occur through divorce, if the non-custodial parent leaves and doesn't maintain a relationship with the child. The inward impression of the child is, "I must have been bad to make Daddy [or Mommy] go away and leave me."

The loss of a parent cannot be understood by a child. Grief goes unexpressed because a child doesn't know how to acknowledge the loss and express it. Insecurity may result from the loss, making fertile ground for depression. Repressed anger may also be present. The child is angry at God for taking his parent away. Trauma is inevitable for a child who loses a parent prematurely. That trauma, if unresolved, makes fertile ground for growing depression in the adult years.

LEARNED PATTERN OF DEPRESSION

In the early years of our life, without any deliberate attempt on our part, we copy our parents' behavior patterns. We especially copy the patterns of the parent of the same sex. We automatically "take in" his or her behavior. If our parents had a problem with depression, we might have identified with them in such a way as to imitate their depressive reaction to life.

> . . . Depression is learned as a way of life. It is learned as a way to handle stress. Depressed families can pass the depressive lifestyle from one generation to the next and to the next. Children do identify with parents and do become like them in their personalities and in the way they handle stressful situations. . . . Individuals who spend their entire childhood identifying with negativistic, chronically depressed parents are going to learn similar attitudes. . . .[7]

If an adult woman has a problem with depression, without an obvious cause such as a recent loss, then her problem may be one of a learned response. If it is, the depressive response will be difficult to eradicate from her life; but it can be done. It's not impossible. It will take a recognition of where the problem is coming from and a strong determination to try to change a learned response.

The effects of uncaring parents, lack of a mother's love, lack of a father's affirmation, loss of a parent, and learned behavior response are deep roots of depression. They have been buried deep within us for a long time.

> During the first five or six years of life, when the basis of personality is formed, thousands of incidents and emotions are recorded and filed away. More than ninety-nine percent of all that transpires in those earliest years is buried in the unconscious mind; but those feelings and reactions are all affecting each of us every moment of our lives. The way we react to a given situation at age thirty or forty was largely determined in the first five years of life.[8]

This doesn't mean that our past dooms us to a life of depression. It simply means that the deep sources of our vulnerability *may* go back to the early years of our life. Consequently, the struggle for some of us to live a positive life may be harder than for others who had early positive influences; but it can be done.

Uncaring parents, lack of a mother's love, lack of a father's affirmation, loss of a parent, and learned behavior patterns are outside influences from our past. We had no control over what happened to us. Now, let's look at some things from our past which we are more directly responsible for. These things may also contribute to our vulnerability to depression.

UNFINISHED BUSINESS

Maggie Scarf says no one reaches the shores of maturity without having taken on a "freightload of unresolved issues." In her book on depression, she calls those unresolved issues "unfinished business."

> Somewhere, lost in . . . women's histories, was a problem left unsolved, a growing-task never completed, a psychological bill left unpaid; important business that had been avoided or evaded, but never really transacted, never completed. . . .[9]

What are some of the unresolved issues affecting the lives of women, making them vulnerable to depression? Let's look at the ones Maggie Scarf mentioned.

1. Uncompleted growing tasks. Good mental health means that we work through the issues of the growing stages of our lives—adolescence, the twenties, the thirties, the middle years, and the later years. It means the tasks of each segment were worked through as we moved freely into the next stage. If they weren't, later we can get bogged down. We can be depressed about something at thirty-five that we should have dealt with when we were twenty.

For example, some women never really achieve a healthy separation from home base. A healthy separation means that a woman lives in terms of meeting her own goals and setting her own standards. An unhealthy separation means she is still trying to please her parents. She lacks an inner confidence to make it on her own. She can't move freely into the future because she can't give up the past. She tends to drag fragments of the tie that once bound her so powerfully to her parents and siblings forward into her adult life.

2. A psychological bill left unpaid. An adult woman can be depressed because of an incestuous incident or several incidents she had as a child with her father or some other male family member. Such an incident is usually packed with anger and guilt. Anger—how could *he* do such a thing to me! Guilt—how could *I* have participated in such a thing! With her adult mind, she holds herself responsible even though she was a child at the time. One woman told me, "The memory of what my father did to me is always with me. I am never free. I try to drown myself in church work to keep from thinking about it, but it always comes back."

3. Important business that has been evaded. Holding grudges indicates unfinished business. These grudges can be deeply buried. We may be ashamed or afraid to admit them, even to ourselves, so they have lain smoldering for years. We have gone way beyond the sin of holding grudges past sundown (Ephesians 4:26). We nursed them for months and even years, until the resentments raised their ugly heads in the form of depression. We must be careful at this point. We may be tempted to look for face-saving reasons for our depression—such as hypoglycemia or hormones—rather than admit to unfinished business in our lives.

4. Problems left unsolved. Loss of believing in God's purpose for our lives caused my first depression. The depression was so miserable, I worked my way out of it by concentrating on a book deadline and several exciting speaking engagements.

A year later, with the book and the speaking engagements behind me, I became depressed again. When my doctor hinted that I might be depressed, I assured him I didn't have any reason to be. Bob was doing well in his job. Our children were well and reasonably contented. I had some interesting writing projects coming up. My future looked good, but I was miserable, more miserable than I had been in my first depression.

I did have physical problems, so the doctor let me have my way (that time!) about not being depressed. He treated me for the physical problems, and I got better. Physically I was all right; but I still felt miserable. Perhaps, I had to admit, part of my problem was emotional. Alone, on my daily walk, I prayed, "God, if my illness is emotional, show me."

Later that day, all the clutter of the first depression surfaced. I realized I was still grieving over what had happened to us. I was still angry over the way some Christians had treated us; and more than that, I still didn't believe God had a purpose for us. When the clutter surfaced, I knew God had answered my prayer, showing me the toll that unfinished business was taking in my life.

I was astonished. Up until that point in my life, I had never realized what an effect the subconscious could have on the physical and how hidden one's emotional hurts could be. While I had adamantly insisted to the doctor that I had no reason to be depressed, there were plenty of reasons inside, working furiously, to make me ill. The excitement and motivation of writing and speaking had covered them up but had not eliminated them. They were still there for me to face.

In a way, those of us who have a problem of unfinished business seem to know about it the least. We seem to be able to make no connection between our present unhappiness and unresolved issues from the past. But unfinished business is there, having its effect on our lives, making us vulnerable to depression. Our recovery may necessitate giving up our relentless examination of surface causes and being willing to look beneath the surface for unfinished business. Is there an old problem left unsolved? Has important business been avoided? Is there a psychological bill left unpaid? Is there an incompleted growing task?

Through looking at the past—both that which we were responsible for and that which we weren't—we can understand that the roots of depression can be very long and can grow very deep. Tough gardening will be needed to eradicate the roots, but it can be done. Just realizing the roots are there is an appropriate place to begin. The past may make us vulnerable to depression or even cause depression, as in the case of unfinished business; but it does not doom us to a future of depression.

[1]Minirth and Meier, *op. cit.*, p. 47.
[2]*Ibid.*, p. 52.
[3]LaHaye, *op. cit.*, p. 50.
[4]Scarf, *op. cit.*, p. 74.
[5]*Ibid.*, p. 73.
[6]Osborne, *op. cit.*, p. 63.
[7]Minirth and Meier, *op. cit.*, p. 108.
[8]Osborne, *op. cit.*, pp. 65-6.
[9]Scarf, *op. cit.*, p. 22.

EIGHT
HOW A WOMAN'S BODY AFFECTS DEPRESSION

When we looked at the causes of depression, we learned that loss, hidden feelings, exhaustion, and so forth cause depression. We also learned that a woman's nature, her world, the times in which she lives, and her past may make her vulnerable to depression. All of these things have to do with thoughts and feelings; they trigger depression. The resulting depression brings about physical changes: sleep patterns change, the appetite changes, constipation and unidentifiable illnesses occur. In this way, the mind affects the body. What is happening inwardly causes physiological changes.

But the reverse is also true. The body affects the mind. Some physiological changes bring about depression or a vulnerability to depression. In chapter one, we learned that both men and women are susceptible to depressive feelings with the onslaught of some physical problems such as the flu. Now we want to see how a woman's body in particular may contribute to depression or depressive feelings.

While there are subtle physical differences in men and women (the way we use our brains is one), the most obvious difference lies in the reproductive role. The woman is the one who has the baby! We want to examine woman's reproductive role to see if her uniqueness contributes to her vulnerability to depression. Let's look at menstruation, pregnancy, postpartum, lactation, and menopause to see which of these areas may be conducive to depression and why.

MENSTRUATION

Have you ever felt especially vulnerable and blue and couldn't fathom why? Perhaps you thought, "How could a born-again, Spirit-filled Christian who practices daily devotions have such blue days?" If these thoughts occurred the week prior to your menstrual period, then you have experienced the effect of the body upon the mind.

In between a woman's menstrual periods, hormonal changes are taking place. The estrogens and progesterone are very active, rising and falling in different proportions to regulate ovulation. Before ovulation occurs, the estrogens are dominant. They are in the process of increasing until they peak at ovulation. After ovulation, progesterone is dominant. The estrogens peak again during this time, but progesterone remains dominant.

Some four or five days before menstruation, progesterone takes a steep, abrupt nose dive. Estrogens, at the same time, are also falling rapidly, but not with the same steep sharpness. Some experts believe that this sudden hormone withdrawal makes women susceptible to depression and to depressive feelings and other disturbances right before their periods. Other experts believe the disturbances are "... caused by a hormonal or hormonally related imbalance, a misstep in the complex minuet of progesterone, estrogen and other chemicals that regulate menstruation."[1]

The drop in progesterone is particularly suspect as the cause because of its sedative action. Progesterone is known as the "quieting" hormone. It appears to have some natural analgesic effects. It acts as an internally produced sedative, providing a calming influence on behavior. It's like being on a sedative for awhile, and then having it suddenly withdrawn.

This sudden hormone withdrawal is thought to be the cause of the mood changes, headaches, tension, anxiety, water retention, irritability, cramping, and so forth that a large number of women experience right before their periods. There are many symptoms and they vary from woman to woman. They also include headaches (migraines), abdominal bloating, change in sleeping patterns, acne, tenderness and swelling of the breasts, mood swings, dizziness, constipation, less frequent urination, and craving for sweets.

Not all women experience these premenstrual symptoms. Some women have mild symptoms; some women have severe symptoms. And 10 percent of women experience severe cases, while milder symptoms affect as many as 40 to 60 percent of all women.[2]

Of those who do suffer, no one woman will experience all the symptoms. Different women are affected in different ways. One doctor who has heavily researched this area classifies the symptoms by groups. Two of the groups have depression as a symptom. In one group, depressive feelings are characteristic. In another group, depression can be so severe as to be life threatening. A woman may have suicidal thoughts and even attempt suicide. She may be tempted to hit her children or ask her husband for a divorce. One fine Christian woman said, "All month long I am a good mother, patient with my children; but right before my period, I feel like whacking them up against the wall."

Some doctors have given labels to these symptoms occurring right before menstruation. Some call it PMT for premenstrual tension. Others call it PMS for premenstrual syndrome. PMT or PMS is not to be confused with menstrual cramps. That's another problem! PMT or PMS is not something a woman outgrows; it worsens with age. This doesn't mean we should have a pessimistic outlook about our future or feel doomed because of it. When we understand what is happening, we are better able to deal with it.

A woman needs to keep a menstrual calendar, keeping track of the days when she experiences physical and emotional changes. If a pattern develops with the same symptoms happening almost every month before her period, she needs to recognize this time as one of vulnerability for her. If a woman's symptoms are very severe (suicidal thoughts, for example), she needs to seek medical help. For many of us, recognizing the pattern is enough to help us deal with it. Becoming aware and accepting the fact that there are days when we are less tolerant and more irritable will enable us to cope. We are biological creatures; changes within our body do affect our moods.

PREGNANCY

A woman is *more* susceptible to depressive feelings prior to menstruation than she normally is. She is *less* likely to be depressed while she is pregnant than she normally is.

Female hormones are present in generous and ever increasing amounts in a woman's body throughout pregnancy. The estrogens and progesterone are being churned out at high levels. At birth, some of the estrogens are some one hundred times higher than they are during the last half of the menstrual cycle. Another estrogen is present at about one thousand times higher than during ordinary menstrual fluctuations. Progesterone is also being produced in highly enlarged quantities. During the last three months of pregnancy, a woman's progesterone level has risen some tenfold from what it is during the second half of her menstrual cycle. The level is about sixty-five times higher than when she is in the first half of the menstrual cycle.

Related to the generous supply of hormones is a feeling of enhanced well-being. This sense of feeling good is due to the increasing levels of the "quieting" hormone, progesterone. This is a time of low vulnerability to depression.

There is a decreased risk of mental illness among females who are pregnant.

Women are less likely to develop a psychiatric disturbance while they are pregnant. The risk of mental illness is lowered during the latter months of pregnancy, when the expectant mother's hormones are circulating through the bloodstream at such high levels. For maladapted and neurotic women, the months of pregnancy are frequently a time of feeling surprisingly good.

I was awed in this study of women and depression as I saw how love bonding works and how progesterone works. It's an awesome thing to see how we as women are responding to God's design and forethought. God planned and designed for survival of life, and progesterone plays a part in that. It keeps the mother calm, providing the proper setting for the fetus to grow. It also prevents the uterus from undergoing its ordinary, rather violent contractions. If those uterine muscles were contracting, as they do as a matter of course, expulsion of the fetus would be far more likely to occur. Progesterone quiets the uterine muscles. At the same time, it is exercising a mildly tranquilizing effect upon the mother's behavior.

POSTPARTUM

In contrast to the general well-being of pregnancy, postpartum is a time of enhanced vulnerability to mental disturbance. The term postpartum refers to one of three general time frames: the first ten days after giving birth, the first three months after giving birth, or the first six months.

The first ten days after childbirth is a time of high emotionality and unusual fragility for many women. Some two thirds of postpartum psychiatric reactions (often depression) occur in this time span.

> But an enhanced vulnerability to mental disturbance seems to extend well beyond that small ten-day span. For, as the

> statistics illustrate with great clarity, new mothers are at a greatly increased risk—some *four* or *five* times greater—of developing a psychological illness in the first three months after delivery. For the entire first six months after having given birth, moreover, the woman who's engaged in early mothering is far more "at risk" for the development of some psychiatric disorder than are women in general.[3]

The emotional fragility that occurs during postpartum is sometimes referred to as "the baby blues." The baby blues aren't experienced only by women who already happen to be maladjusted or psychologically unsteady. Research indicates that there's a difference during this time even for ordinarily stable and well-functioning women. Following the birth of the baby, there is an abrupt drop in levels of different endocrine agents that have been circulating in a woman's plasma. This is a biologically induced state similar to what happens to a person coming off drugs. In this case, it is a female-hormone withdrawal.

This dramatic decline in hormone levels is the same thing that happens four or five days before menstruation; only the drop is *much* greater at this time. At labor's onset, two of the estrogens are present at levels that are about one hundred times higher than they are in the second phase of the menstrual cycle. At the time of birth, these estrogens drop dramatically and make a slow return to non-pregnancy levels. Another estrogen is present just before labor at one thousand times higher than during the second phase of the menstrual cycle. After delivery, the estrogens don't return to normal for anywhere from two weeks to twenty-one days.

As for progesterone, the pregnant woman has been synthesizing it at the rate of about two hundred to three hundred milligrams per day. This is ten times higher, on a daily basis, than what she produces during the second half of her menstrual cycle.

> After the birth of her child her progesterone levels will be so vastly lowered that they could be termed negligible to the point of nonexistence. And the enhanced risk of mental illness in the postpartum period very probably reflects what is a suddenly and drastically altered internal hormonal status, for these are truly very ample and impressive biochemical changes and shifts.[4]

What are the symptoms of this female-hormone withdrawal? The new mother is moody and irritable; her moods tend to swing up and down more easily than usual. She is uncommonly prone to crying. She might experience unusual fears or worries. She might be afraid she'll die. She may worry over her ability to adequately care for her new baby. She will experience depressive feelings, and she may become clinically depressed. Not knowing what is happening to her, she may blame the emotional way she is feeling on someone else—particularly her husband.

The new mother may be extraordinarily prone to identifying with others during postpartum. She is unusually empathetic. These feelings of empathy are very much needed for new mothering. To feel for another is very important to being a good mother. Empathetic feelings are needed to meet the baby's needs—a baby who can be demanding and unpredictable.

In order to manage the baby blues and to attempt to meet the baby's needs, there's nothing wrong with saying, "I need help." In today's society, it's considered normal that a woman fresh from delivery be thrown under heavy stress, be expected to work as hard or harder than she ever has, and do it all on less sleep than normal. Self-sufficiency is so inculcated in the American woman that she thinks she is a bad mother for not being able to meet all of her baby's and her husband's needs during this period. Today's mother thinks she isn't supposed to need help.

A woman having her baby today may never have been

exposed to the day-by-day care of an infant, so she has no idea of what to expect. Neither is she going to benefit from the experience of other women in the family, because she may be living hundreds of miles away from them. Up until World War I, a new mother commonly went straight home to her mother with a new baby. In many communities all the neighbor women pitched in. A new mother was treated like a queen bee. What a wonderful idea! As a new mother learned to meet the needs of her child, other women came to her aid. Research suggests that a woman who receives real support right from the birth of her baby (and not just lip service—"If you need anything, be sure to let me know") is less likely to suffer severe or prolonged postpartum depression.

LACTATION

The latest research is now *suggesting* that there may be built-in help for the new mother if she nurses her baby. One of the major hormones associated with nursing, prolactin, may have the same analgesic, sedating effects as does progesterone. Both of these hormones seem to provide the mother with some biochemical protection against stress. Both seem to work toward influencing the pregnant or nursing woman toward a more quiescent state of being.

The biological equipment God gave to pregnant mothers protects the baby and makes the mother feel good at the same time. The equipment of nursing mothers, research is suggesting, enables women to be in tune with signals coming from their babies and to be less responsive to all of the other things going on in her environment. God designed women to provide for the preservation of life.

MENOPAUSE

Menopause marks the cessation of menstruation and the end of a woman's reproductive ability. It rarely is experienced as an event that can be pinpointed in time. Menopause takes place in a nebulous fashion and happens over a period of anywhere from several months to several years. Technically, menopause has been accomplished when a woman has gone through an entire year without a period. Once a woman has gone through that year without any bleeding, she's considered to have completed her cycles.

In the past, menopause usually occurred in the late forties. "With increased life expectancy and improved health among U.S. women, menopause now occurs, on the average, after 50."[5]

Menopause does involve hormonal change. Changes in the levels of the estrogens and progesterone begin long before any obvious signs of menopause become evident. Long before a female's periods have become irregular or have ceased, her reproductive hormone production has been slowing down. The decline is gradual, not a sudden dip as with premenstruation and postpartum.

There has been a strong tendency to correlate the declining of the hormones associated with menopause with depression. Even many experts claim a cause and effect association between the depressed female and the status of her reproductive system. However, recent scientific research reports no connection of menopausal hormonal decline as the cause of depression during the middle years. We do see a correlation between vulnerability to depression during premenstruation and postpartum, but both of those involve a sudden, steep drop in hormones.

The idea that menopause provides a biological reason for depression during the middle years is a tenaciously held belief. Contrary to the latest research, the powerful belief in a change-of-life depression will probably continue to exist. It sounds right to most people, even to people who should know better.

An acquaintance of mine was struggling with depression the same time I was. Her doctor's diagnosis was, "You're experiencing an early menopause." She was thirty-eight. It is always going to be easier to diagnose a woman's depression as biological than go to the effort to find out what the real cause is.

If menopause rendered a woman far more depression prone, wouldn't there be more depression among women in this age group? There isn't. The rates of depression are higher among women in their early thirties.

This is not to say that women can't and don't get depressed during the years between forty-five and fifty-five. A woman may, but her condition will be a result of other disruptive events such as those of the middle years mentioned in chapter six. Her depression will not be caused by her declining hormones.

Women need to know that there are some physical changes associated with menopause that are disturbing. These are hot flushes (sometimes called hot flashes) and "night sweats"—flushes occurring at night. They are not imagined; they really occur, in some degree, to a majority of women. Both are directly related to estrogen loss.

> With the decline in hormonal secretions, neurovascular control becomes very labile. The blood vessels seem to over-respond to tiny temperature shifts—which may be caused by anger, excitement, being in a crowd, or simply by having one blanket too many. In short, there is a deficiency in the mechanisms regulating heat loss. The red face or bath of sweat that can result from a minor heat change would be more appropriate to a vast temperature change: the woman's body is responding as though she's not just slightly warmer, but as though she's in the midst of the Sahara![6]

Night sweats and hot flushes are clearly associated with menopause, but a *biologically* initiated depression is not associated with this phase of female life.

The purpose of this chapter has been to see when we are vulnerable to depression for biological reasons. Premenstruation and postpartum, both limited periods of time, are times of more susceptibility than usual for many women. Pregnancy and perhaps nursing are times of lessened vulnerability. The hormonal withdrawal associated with menopause does not cause depression. Understanding these things should help us live with ourselves.

Understanding should also help us see that God's design for woman includes a system that can be trusted for the survival of life. This system, though, does leave a woman with times of need—right before her menstrual period and right after giving birth. Times of need don't have to be times for berating ourselves on how incapable we are. Times of need can be times of blessing as we also acknowledge our need for spiritual refreshment and for supportive companionship. Letting others minister to us can be a real blessing.

Understanding is also a freeing experience. It sets us free from the bondage of the unknown, of suspecting that the biological system God gave us is playing sinister tricks on us. Understanding sets free forces of strength and insight within us, enabling us to cope. What a woman understands, she can handle.

[1]Natalie Angier with Janet Witzleben, "Dr. Jekyll and Ms. Hyde," *Reader's Digest*, February, 1983, p. 121. ©1982 DISCOVER Magazine, Time Inc. Reprinted with permission.
[2]*Ibid.*, p. 120.
[3]Scarf, *op. cit.*, p. 277.
[4]*Ibid.*, p. 286.
[5]Matt Clark and Mariana Gosnell, "Managing the Menopause," *Newsweek*, February 9, 1981, Vol. 97, p. 92.
[6]Scarf, *op. cit.*, pp. 404, 405.

NINE
GETTING OVER DEPRESSION REQUIRES SELF-HELP

In this book, we have gained an understanding of the illness of depression and an understanding of why women are vulnerable to it. A third thing we need to understand is how to fight depression.

The best ammunition we can have in fighting depression is the knowledge that we will probably win the fight. For any given case of depression that a woman experiences, there is a 95 percent chance of recovery.

Depression is a self-lifting illness. Most cases of depression eventually disappear without treatment. If given enough time, things will correct themselves. The miserable feelings, the hopelessness, the agony will be left behind. If this wasn't true, human history might have been very different. Abraham Lincoln, Nathaniel Hawthorne, Winston Churchill, and astronaut Buzz Aldrin are all accomplished people who have had recurrent bouts of depression. They managed to ride through their depressions, and we can, too. No depression lasts forever. Ours will eventually come to an end.

If depression is self-lifting and has a high recovery rate, then it seems ironical that we are going to need to spend the next three chapters on how to fight depression. (To spend less than that is to underestimate the enemy.) The knowledge that we will win should give us hope and courage, but not make us naive about what we are struggling with. There are some very good reasons why we ought to try to get over depression.

1. Not to try to get over depression is to take a chance on doing something that will be regretted later when the depression lifts. In chapter two we saw how many of the symptoms of depression have to do with a person's thinking patterns. The thinking patterns of a depressed person are distorted. Because of this distortion, depressed persons sometimes make disastrous mistakes while they are depressed. They have even gone so far as to quit their job or walk out of their marriage. When the depression lifts, they look back and think, "How could I have ever done such a thing?"

2. Not to try to get over depression is to set ourselves up for more hurt. This is called the "depressive theorem." Feeling bad seems to bring about situations in which bad things happen. These bad events then serve to deepen our depression, to confirm the many rotten things we already knew about ourselves. This can be traced to a depressed woman's lessened ability to cope and to be flexible; her actions are not what they should be. Or, the feelings of inability could be on an unconscious level; we unconsciously set ourselves up to prove how awful we are or how bad our situation is. Either way, the unwelcomed sequelae or secondary effects that follow our depression really hurt. Not to get over our depression is to set ourselves up for unnecessary—and often hard-to-forget—hurts.

3. Not to try to get over depression is to set ourselves up for chronic or habitual depression, in which depression becomes a way of responding to life's disappointments. This is what I was afraid was happening to me. My three depressions took place within two years. A year divided

the first two, but the third one came in a matter of a few months after the second one. A pattern was beginning in which my response to life's disappointments was a depressive one.

Or, some experts would say I had chronic depression. In chronic depression, a person pulls herself out of a depression just far enough that the physical symptoms are eliminated. She starts sleeping better. Her appetite returns to normal. The stomach pains cease. Feeling physically good again enables her to go on with her work but it doesn't necessarily mean she has eliminated the negative view of life that comes with depression. Consequently, she develops a depressive outlook on life. It is a cheerless, hopeless outlook that always expects the worst. Rigorous self-control is needed to keep from succumbing to chronic depression.

4. Not to try to get over depression is to set ourselves up for suicidal tendencies. If the illness of depression lingers, going unchecked, it can lead to hopelessness, making life nothing but a horrible nightmare. All a depressed person can remember are moments of suffering; the good moments are blotted out. All of this would be bearable if she had the conviction that things would eventually improve. The hopelessness of depression makes a woman think things never will improve. She sees the future as holding only more pain and turmoil.

We must never underestimate what these feelings of hopelessness will do to us. Research studies show that an unrealistic sense of hopelessness is one of the most crucial factors in the development of a serious suicidal wish. Suicide becomes more and more attractive when life appears to be a trap from which there seems to be no escape. Suicide begins to look like the only way of escape.

Bad feelings, self-deprecation, hopelessness, and suicide are part of the spiraling effects of depression. Not to try to get over depression is to take a chance of being caught in the spiral. Depression is the only psychiatric disorder which has a high mortality rate: 95 percent of depressants do recover, but as many as 5 percent commit suicide.

These four reasons for trying to get over depression show us the seriousness of our situation. If we don't want to make regrettable mistakes, if we don't want unnecessary hurts, if we don't want to make our depression habitual or be tempted to commit suicide, then we need to know how to fight depression.

WHAT'S ESSENTIAL TO GETTING WELL

There is no one way in to depression, and there is no one way out. Despite the similarity of symptoms of depressed people, they're not alike in how they got that way, and they do not get over it in the same way. Every woman who has recovered from depression has her story to tell. The details of each woman's story differ, but underneath the details are two basic essentials—essentials that even she may not be aware of. The two essentials are admitting we have depression and wanting to get over it.

We don't like to admit we have a problem, but that's exactly what we must do. We have to accept responsibility for our depression. It doesn't matter who wronged us, how unjust they were, or how unfair life is—the depression is ours. We are responsible for our depressive reaction, and our admittance is the key for setting ourselves free.

Our admittance that we have a problem doesn't take away the guilt of the person or persons who wronged us; but that's their problem. Depression is ours, and the sooner we admit it, the sooner we will be on our way to recovery. A famous psychologist said that he considers only one kind of counselee relatively hopeless. It's the person who blames other people for her problems. If we can own the mess we're in, he says, then there is hope and help available. As long as we blame others, we'll be victims of our depression.

Most of us hate to face up to our human responsibility,

especially when it comes to our own emotional state. Many women have been depressed for weeks or months and knew it, but kept thinking, "I should be able to get this under control. In a day or two, I'll be able to handle it."

Oh, how it hurts to admit we have a problem. It may help by saying out loud, "I am depressed." We may need to say it over and over again, until we've admitted the fact to ourselves.

If that doesn't help, we should tell someone. Say to a close friend, "I'm having a problem with depression." This confession will exteriorize our problem and help us gain outside support. Telling someone else will also ignite our self-will and encourage us to try harder.

Once we have admitted we are depressed, we need to ask ourselves, do we really *want* to get well? Wanting to get well is essential to getting over depression, and here are some reasons why.

1. Fighting depression is tough. When people ask me how I finally got over depression, my answer is SHEER GRIT. They look shocked because I know they expect to hear a story of supernatural delivery. Supernatural help came in time, but not until I was determined to get well. The sides of the pit of depression I was in were slippery and slimy. I would make some progress up the side and then slide back again. When my fingers reached the top of the pit, something would happen to cause me to lose my grip, and I would slide back down. What sent me back down the side didn't have to be anything major. Things that wouldn't have bothered me under normal circumstances became devastating events that impeded my progress. It took a lot of work to get out of the pit and stay out.

David Ray, an evangelist who also had trouble with depression said, "If it meant . . . starting all over again, that was a price I was willing to pay to win the war I was involved in. I had to swallow every ounce of pride I ever had and I had more than my share. Many were the days when I had to shove my shoulders back and push my head up and say, 'I will not give up. I will win this war.' And I won."[1]

2. Another reason why we must want to get well is because of the continuity needed. Our progress in getting well may not rise steadily. It may be a complicated path with dips and drops in it.

Getting over depression does not look like this.

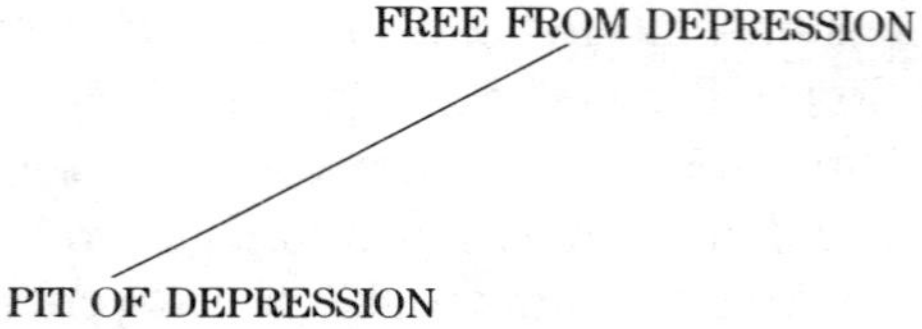

Figure 1

Recovery looks more like this.

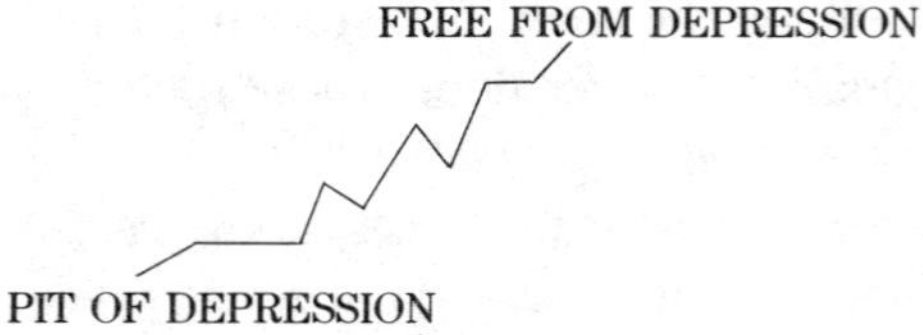

Figure 2

There will be days when we will feel so bad, we'll decide that we are no better. But even at the bottom of the dips we are higher than we were. We'll have enough symptom-free hours and even days that will make us believe the bad days will eventually disappear—until we are well again.

3. Depression can have a powerful hold on us. We must want to get well in order to break that hold. Depression can begin to feel very comfortable. There's a certain satisfaction in feeling sorry for ourselves. (After all, we reason, nobody else does!) Depression can even begin to feel normal. We hold onto it like an old bathrobe or a favorite pair of tennis shoes. Nobody in the world can take it away from us! We must not underestimate the power of depression. We must want to get rid of it.

4. Depression can also be power for us. We never really intend for this to happen, but it is part of the subtlety of depression. A woman begins with a simple depression over a loss or disappointment; and then, in the misery of her symptoms, she sees that the depression has an effect on others. Every one in the family tries harder to please her. Or, the gals in the Sunday school class call more often. Or, the girls at the office are eager to help with the extra typing. Our depression influences the behavior of others. If we like their response, we may be tempted to keep the depression or at least let it come back periodically.

Or, the depression may serve as a way of keeping our loss alive. One women I talked with had lost her six-year-old son in tragic, freakish circumstances. She was depressed over his death for four years. She said, "As long as I was depressed, Sonny was alive." Her symptoms kept his memory alive.

These four reasons should help us see how much we need to want to get over depression. It's imperative to getting well. Dr. David Burns says, "Many depressed individuals will go through a phase in which they *stubbornly refuse* to do anything to help themselves. The moment this crucial motivational problem has been solved, the depression typically begins to diminish. . . ."[2] We must admit we are depressed and we must want to get well if we are going to climb out of the pit of depression and win the war.

HELPS FOR GETTING OVER DEPRESSION

Once we have admitted we have depression and want to get well, we need tools to help us make the steep ascent out of the pit of depression. Because the ascent is slippery and slimy, we may need a pick and a rope or a ladder—some tools to help us make progress. Not everyone uses the same tools. Here is a list of tools that come recommended by those who have recovered from depression or who have helped others recover.

1. *Take a good look at your depression.* You have already reached for a tool by reading this book. Now that you know something about depression and its causes, it's time to take a good look at yours. See if you can identify a cause. What loss have you experienced? Have you moved recently? Has someone close to you died? Has a dear friend moved away? Are you having trouble at work? What illnesses have you developed? With whom have you been angry? Who has disappointed you? Have you experienced changes involving a lot of stress over the last eighteen months?

If you can pinpoint the cause, you might want to relax and trust in the fact that it will pass. One psychologist recommends going with the symptoms rather than fighting them. Depression is going to lift, so the symptoms are going to pass. The best tactic then is to go with the symptoms. Take it easy for awhile. A brief time out from your responsibilities, if you can take time out, or a slowing down of activity may be beneficial. Trying to disguise your feelings and carrying on like a superwoman will only make the depression worse. Remember when God responded to Elijah's depression, he started at his most basic level of need with food and rest (1 Kings 19:5-8).

Depressive illnesses usually last from four months to a year. That will help you judge approximately where you are as far as the progress of the illness and whether you want to wait it out.

If you *cannot* pinpoint the cause or if you have had repeated depressive episodes, do not try this approach. Some of the other tools might be better for you as well as the help to be prescribed in the next chapter.

2. *Talk to someone you trust.* The Bible says, "Confess *your* faults one to another, and pray one for another, that ye may be healed . . ." (James 5:16a). Talking out our feelings has good therapeutic value and helps us exteriorize our problems. If we can see our problems outside of ourselves, they may look altogether different. To keep them

inside is to risk distorting them. Talking clears out all those inward things such as unexpressed anger or unresolved guilt that are causing our depression. Great relief will come in just talking about what's bothering us. Talking will also engage the help and prayerful support of the other person, removing the loneliness of our illness.

Talking with just anybody will not do. If we pick the wrong person, we may end up more depressed! We need a good listener—one who doesn't continually interrupt with her own experiences, who can keep confidences, who will not be shocked or judgmental, and who is not equipped with ready answers. That kind of listener is rare!

Dr. Roy W. Fairchild in his book on counseling depressed persons recommends looking for a "wounded healer." In our case, a wounded healer would be a fellow Christian who has experienced deep sorrow in life and recovered. The wounded healer does not have ready quips for life's deep hurts. A wounded healer knows it's listening that you need, not instant remedies.

If you cannot find a trusted friend or fellow church member to listen to you, talking out your feelings is still going to be helpful. Look for a counselor. Your pastor may be a counselor. Make an appointment to talk with him, or ask him to refer you to a counselor. Look for a mental health clinic in your area. For a directory of federally funded mental health centers, write to the National Institute of Mental Health, 5600 Fishers Lane, Rockville, MD 20857.

While waiting for an appointment with a counselor or in addition to seeing a counselor, you might want to talk out your feelings with God in the person of his Son Jesus. Imagine Jesus' presence with you—across the table, at the opposite end of the couch, or in the next chair. You don't actually have to put a face to your imaginative figure. You simply need a mental image to help you consciously acknowledge Jesus' presence.

Out loud (this is a must!), you might want to say something like this, "Jesus, I'm glad you are here with me. I need a good listener, someone to understand what I am going through. I know you do. You were rejected by your friends, and there was even a time when you felt abandoned by God. That's the way I've felt lately. Sometimes I think God has forgotten all about me. You see I've been terribly hurt and disappointed. I'm angry and mad and confused. I need your help." Then proceed to tell him your feelings as you would a trusted friend.

In this kind of praying, you are not asking for a direct answer. Answers and solutions are not what you need at this point. You need a listener to help you get your feelings out from within. There is great relief in externalizing our problems. Talking with a trusted friend, whether that be someone in the flesh or Jesus, is probably the best tool we can use in getting over depression.

3. *Get moving.* If depression is making you drag around and causing you not to want to get out of bed in the morning, you need to take action. Movement will make you less depressed. Dr. David Burns says that virtually any meaningful activity has a chance of brightening our mood.

> If you do nothing, you will become preoccupied with the flood of negative, destructive thoughts. If you do something, you will be temporarily distracted from that internal dialogue of self-denigration. What is even more important, the sense of mastery you will experience will disprove many of the distorted thoughts that slowed you down in the first place.[3]

Don't wait until you feel like doing something in the way of desire or energy. You might never get moving if you do! You must make yourself get moving—take a brisk walk, go jogging, biking, swimming, or play tennis. Even a good scrubbing of the kitchen floor might be stimulation enough to fight the immobilization of depression.

4. *Set small goals for yourself.* Self-esteem is enhanced by setting goals and reaching them. Too often, depressives

feel hopeless and worthless, incapable of reaching any goal. We can fight the hopelessness by setting small goals that are realistic. For a starter, the goal may be as simple as "OK, I'm going to get out of bed today by nine o'clock." The next day, our goal might be to be out of bed, dressed, and have the dishes washed by nine o'clock. Accomplishing even minor tasks will help us realize we can function, that we are not helpless and that we have more strength than we think we do.

When you're depressed, inertia has a real edge on you. You have a heightened awareness of the absurdity of life, which will make you wonder if there's any point in going on. Every goal will appear to demand too much and will seem not to be worth the trouble. But if you go ahead, set a realistic goal and reach it, it will boost your self-esteem.

5. *Give yourself pleasure.* One psychotherapist suggests buying yourself a small present, perhaps new lipstick or a new pair of earrings—something just for you. Maybe you could give yourself pleasure in the way of a treat—having a new haircut or hiring a baby-sitter for a couple of hours so that you might do something you've been wanting to do. One woman who was depressed over the death of her brother scheduled a personal "retreat" each week. Often this "retreat" was no more than strolling on a favorite pine trail in a nature preserve, but she found it especially gratifying.

Giving yourself pleasure is not a matter of pampering yourself. It's a way of making positive deposits in your emotional bank. We can't always be giving out unless we are sometimes taking in.

6. *Be with other people.* Isolation feeds depression, so it's important not to cut yourself off from social contacts. Isolation deepens the feeling that no one cares. Join a group of some kind, maybe a Bible study group, a craft class, or an exercise class. To be effective, the group needs to be one in which there will be involvement and interaction with other people.

7. *Help someone else.* Self-pity is deadly to the depressed person. To make self the center of our attention is self-destructive. It traps our depression. One way to break out of the trap is to think of other people. This means to be aware of someone else's needs and try to meet them. An interesting line in the book of Job is, "And the Lord turned the captivity of Job, when he prayed for his friends ..." (Job 42:10a). Our captivity can turn, too, when the center of our attention is drawn away from ourselves and directed toward someone else.

Doing for others takes one's mind off oneself and switches it from negative to positive. It restores self-esteem. It may well change the internal conversation from, "I am not good for anything," to, "I am useful to someone; I can do something effectively."

8. *Act your way out.* Several times in my research I came across a quote that goes something like this, "It is easier to act yourself into a new way of feeling than to feel your way into a new way of acting." In essence, the quote means that external changes in our behavior often precede, rather than follow, internal changes. In other words, make your outward actions appear the way you really want to feel. Act as if you are not depressed!

But, you argue, "I don't feel like doing that," or, "I know it won't do any good." Make yourself. Go to your weekly Bible study group. Smile. Greet everyone. Ask about their children. Ask about their jobs. Really listen to their answers. Make yourself act as if you are not hurting on the inside. In the process, as you get caught up in really listening to what the other women say, you forget your own hurts and see that you can feel better.

9. *Clarify the alternatives.* When you are depressed, you have a tendency to confuse feelings and facts. Your feelings say your situation is hopeless. The future is bleak. You can become trapped by the maze of your own feelings. There's also the fear of making a mistake and compounding the problem. Fear inhibits you from thinking of alternatives to

your situation—when actually there are always alternatives. Some of them may seem pretty bizarre, and you may not like some of them, but there are always alternatives.

Florence Littaur, who has counseled many depressed persons, suggests listing the alternatives no matter how bizarre they may be. She suggests listing them in writing. Then think of the possible consequences of each alternative. What would happen if you did number one? What would happen if you did the second alternative?

Clarifying the alternatives will help you take an objective look at your situation. You might even want to go over these alternatives with a good listener. Then, to get the most benefit from this tool, you need to make a decision about which alternative you are going to follow.

Depressives who feel hopeless never actually are totally hopeless. Clarifying the alternatives helps you see hope. Making a decision will give you a plan of action that will get you moving. And, when you're well, you will be able to look back and see that there were many workable answers to what seemed like an insoluble dilemma.

10. *Get a different perspective.* Cautiously, I would like to suggest changing your circumstances as a help in getting over depression. I say "cautiously" because it is contrary to most advice I read. That advice said you can't change your circumstances, you can only change yourself. I agree with that, in the sense that you can't change your husband's nature or your children's temperament. If they are causing you to be depressed, then you can't very well change your circumstances. You must learn to live with those you love as they are.

But if you can change the circumstances that are depressing you, then make the change. If you don't, considering the way depressives think, you will begin to assume that circumstances are the same everywhere. If it is your job that is depressing, you will think it would be the same wherever you worked. If your church is depressing you, you will begin to think all churches are that way. Women will often stay with a situation they are miserable in rather than risk making someone mad. They will also stay with a miserable situation to avoid the insecurity of looking for a better one.

Changing those depressive circumstances can give you a new lease on life. "Well, there are some good working situations," or, "There are some Christians who think and feel like I do." We can drop that general depressive perspective on life we've developed.

Now, if you can't make a change (it is your husband or the kids who are getting to you), then try to gain a fresh perspective on your situation. Meeting a friend for a long, leisurely lunch, or taking a short trip out of town, or attending a woman's retreat will help. It doesn't have to involve a large amount of time as long as it gives you enough time to take a second look at your situation and gain some inner strength for going back to tackle it.

11. *Praise your way out of depression.* Have you noticed how many of these listed tools have to do with drawing attention away from self? Many of the tools pull your attention away from the depression that is absorbing all of your thoughts. Praising God is another way of doing that.

In *Destined for the Throne,* Paul E. Billheimer says that praise decentralizes the self.

> The worship and praise of God demands a shift of center from self to God. One cannot praise without relinquishing occupation with self. When praise becomes a way of life, the infinitely lovely God becomes the center of worship rather than the bankrupt self. Thus the personality becomes properly integrated and destructive stresses and strains disappear. This results in mental wholeness.[4]

Praise also opens the way for God to come in and to impart his strength. One of the common complaints of Christians who are depressed is how far away they feel from God. Praise is a bridge to God.

> Where there is joyful praise, there He is dynamically and benevolently active. In Psalm 22:3 we are told that God "inhabits the praises" of His people. This means that wherever there is adoration, reverence, and acceptable worship and praise, there He identifies and openly manifests His presence.[5]

Praising God when you are depressed is far from easy. That's what makes it a "sacrifice" of praise. "By him therefore let us offer the sacrifice of praise to God continually, that is, the fruit of our lips, giving thanks to his name" (Hebrews 13:15). Billheimer says that "the fruit of our lips" means that the sacrifice of praise is incomplete until it is expressed. Practically speaking, this means the praise must be said out loud and said as if it is really meant. To make this tool work, you must sacrifice your own judgment about your situation, and relinquish all that attention you've been giving to yourself, and verbally express praise to God.

These eleven tools—and there could be others—will work to help you out of the pit of depression *if* you can admit you are depressed and *if* you want to get well. Warning: You can actually go through the motions of doing these activities and still not make any progress. For example, I never stopped being involved with people during all three of my depressions. I also exercised through them all. The tools themselves are not guarantees to getting over depression. They are handles to help you work your way out.

However, since I've come to see that I am vulnerable to depression, I've found all the tools helpful in staying well. The difference is, my will is now engaged. I don't rely on the same tool every time depressive feelings hit. What works one time doesn't work every time. The important thing is that I do something to tackle the feelings. I want to stay well. For me, with my vulnerability, that will always mean a fight.

For others, tackling depression may not require as much of a fight. If the depression is circumstantial, and the cause can be identified, then you know the depression will go away. You may not need to do anything except wait for it to lift.

For others of us, though, the fight isn't so easy. We won't be able to make it out of the pit of depression without some help. In the next chapter we're going to look at what kind of help is available.

[1]Toby Druin, "Admit It or Not, Ray Says, Everybody 'Hurts' Sometime," *Baptist Standard*, February 11, 1981, p. 4.

[2]Burns, *op. cit.*, p. 83.

[3]*Ibid.*, p. 92.

[4]Paul E. Billheimer, *Destined for the Throne* (Fort Washington, Penn.: Christian Literature Crusade, 1975), p. 118. Taken from copyrighted material used by permission of the Christian Literature Crusade, Fort Washington, Penn. 19034.

[5]*Ibid.*, p. 120.

TEN

GETTING OVER DEPRESSION MAY REQUIRE OUTSIDE HELP

Jesus did not have a formula approach to healing. Sometimes he healed through a spoken word or command (Matthew 8:32; 9:2, 6; 12:13). Sometimes the healing was in his touch (Matthew 9:27-30; 8:3). Sometimes he healed from a distance, when the person wasn't even in his presence (Matthew 15:28; Mark 7:30). One time he put his fingers in a man's ears and used his spit to touch the man's eyes (Mark 7:31-37). Once he simply rebuked the illness (Luke 4:39); and once his being available so someone could touch him was enough (Matthew 9:20-22). Jesus recognized that each person is uniquely different, and he treated them all as such. He had no pat, simplistic solutions to the infirmities of men and women.

Neither do we want to have pat, simplistic solutions to depression. Not all of us are going to be healed from depression in the same manner. In the last chapter, we saw a number of different self-helps that people may use to get over depression. Some of us may need more help than those self-help activities can give. We may need professional help. How do we know when we need outside help?

We need help when we don't know what caused the depression. The black cloud of despair came out of nowhere. The despair is dark and deep; and *in all honesty,* we cannot fathom a cause.

We need help if we are having suicidal thoughts.

We need help if we are having delusional thoughts.

We need help if we can't sleep, or we are losing a serious amount of weight, or we are experiencing severe physical discomfort in which our health may be affected.

We need help if we have had repeated depressive episodes in our life.

We need help when the depression is hurting our marriage, our family, or our job.

We definitely need help if the depression has lasted longer than one year.

A woman fitting any of these conditions needs to consider seeking outside help in getting over her depression. Depression is a treatable illness. While there is not one simple cure that works for everyone, there are a number of treatments available. If one method doesn't bring her out of a depression, another likely will. Any woman suffering from depression needs to know how to get help and what kind of help is available.

FINDING HELP

The best place to begin getting help is with your family doctor. A thorough medical examination is necessary in order to rule out physical causes for your depression. Your fatigue, disturbed sleep, or other symptoms may have a physical origin, so a good medical examination is needed.

If the cause isn't physical, and the doctor diagnoses your problem as clinical depression, then you may want to consider seeking further help from a psychiatrist, psychologist, or trained counselor. If your doctor has a good understanding of depression, he will refer you on. A referral to a therapist should be as routine as would be a referral to a surgeon when you need an operation.

A psychiatrist is a medical doctor who is skilled and

practiced in the treatment of depressive disorders. His job is to delineate between the various kinds and causes of depression and to prescribe accordingly. He will work to immediately reduce the depression and to find the cause. The basic tools he uses to do this are psychotherapy, antidepressants, and electroconvulsive therapy.

Clinical psychologists and psychiatric social workers are also psychotherapists trained in counseling techniques, but they cannot prescribe medical treatment (antidepressants and electroconvulsive therapy). They do work along with psychiatrists, so that when medical help is needed, it can readily be obtained.

PSYCHOTHERAPY

Psychotherapy or counseling is talk therapy. By using words to attack depression, psychotherapists try to help patients recognize their feelings and deal with the events that triggered them. Psychotherapy provides three kinds of help: (1) emotional release, (2) insight, and (3) behavioral change.

In a psychotherapy session, the patient discusses her problems, expressing hostility, fear, guilt, and other emotions with freedom. She releases her emotions. As she "talks out" her problems, other feelings of which she may be totally unaware will come to the surface. This is one benefit of the emotional release.

Another benefit is the cleansing effect emotional release provides. The cleansing of the inner tension and pressure a patient has can enable her to cope. The more she bares her soul in a therapeutic situation, the more release she can experience. The relaxation alone will provide a short-term benefit.

The verbal expression of true emotional feeling is considered essential to effective psychotherapy. Until a patient releases her feelings, the tension and conflict associated with them will block any learning of new, more adjustive attitudes. "Airing" problems with a good psychotherapist can provide long-term benefits in addition to immediate relief when we consider the other two aspects of psychotherapy. Emotional release paves the way for the development of insight and positive action toward the solution of our problems.

As we get our emotional conflicts out into the open where we can see them for what they are, we spontaneously gain insight into our motivations and behavior. The therapist then enhances this insight by appropriately interpreting what has happened and by providing a basis for positive action.

As we gain insight into our problems and the faulty ways in which we have been trying to solve them, we are in a position to make behavioral changes and to attempt appropriate adjustive measures. The therapist helps us see what needs to be done, what our alternatives are, and what the consequences of each alternative would be. The therapist does not make the decision for us, but helps us "walk through" the possible solutions and their consequences.

How does talking it out with a counselor differ from talking it out with a good friend? The counselor has been *trained* in listening and probing. There are over one hundred different types of psychotherapies. A large part of the skill of the psychotherapist is in matching the right psychotherapy to the patient's personal problems and strengths. Some of the more common techniques are questioning, interpretation, and free association. Many therapists use several techniques, even with the same patient. What techniques are used will vary from individual to individual.

ANTIDEPRESSANTS

Because in some people the illness of depression is a *physical* disorder as well as a mental and emotional one, it can then be treated with specific medications. The medicines are called antidepressants or "mood elevating" drugs.

There are a variety of drugs available to trained psychiatrists that can help with different types of depression. Because these need to be carefully monitored for dosage level, possible side effects, and dietary changes, be sure to work closely with your doctor. Medications have helped some, but not all depressed people. Under a psychiatrist's care, they are a viable treatment method.

ELECTROCONVULSIVE THERAPY

While depression is a treatable illness, this doesn't mean everyone who has it can get well through psychotherapy. It doesn't mean that everyone who has it can get well through antidepressants. Psychotherapy works for some. Antidepressants work for others. For some, neither works. For severely depressed people, electroconvulsive therapy (ECT) may be needed.

ECT is a series of brief electrical stimulations of the brain. Scientists don't know why the electric stimulations work; but one theory is that ECT may "restart" sluggish brain cells that play a role in mood.

A brain seizure is evoked by a mini-current. A pulse of electricity lasting a fraction of a second is passed through the head to provoke a seizure. A seizure is evoked by a sophisticated machine six to twelve times over two to four weeks. The series of seizures brings about the improvement.

ECT has been a very controversial treatment, but it does seem to bring some people out of their depressions. Like the use of antidepressant drugs, it requires the careful monitoring of a competent psychiatrist and careful consideration by those involved.

Psychotherapy, antidepressants, and electroconvulsive therapy do not describe all of the possible treatments for depression, but they are the basic ones used by psychiatrists and counselors.

PROBLEMS WITH FINDING HELP

The process we've described here of finding help sounds simple and routine, but for many women, getting help is not that easy. For that reason, we need to look at some of the problems encountered when it comes to getting help. Here are some things to be aware of.

1. We should be careful about seeking help from therapists who are fully committed to one form of therapy exclusively. Drug treatments are helpful in improving the biological symptoms of depression such as sleep and appetite loss. Psychotherapy is helpful in improving a person's social and interpersonal functioning. They both have their place. We should seek a competent psychiatrist who will make a responsible judgment on what is best for us.

Depression is a treatable illness, but it's important to seek treatment from someone who allows for more than one way to recovery. Two patients with what may appear to be identical symptoms might have different underlying disorders, calling for different methods of treatment.

2. We should be cautious about seeking help from a general practitioner alone, as many are not especially trained when it comes to the use of antidepressant drugs. These drugs are powerful medications and need the monitoring of someone with considerable pharmacological skill and know how. They require supervision over time, too, as dosage levels and possible side-effects must be carefully and knowledgeably monitored. General practitioners may know too little about diagnosing the condition and prescribe the wrong drug or offer too little of the correct drug. Antidepressants have to reach therapeutic dosage levels before they can provide any relief.

It would be rare to find a general practitioner with the time and probing skills needed for psychotherapy. This is not to say a general practitioner would not be compassionate and understanding; but psychotherapy involves more than that. Besides, how open would you really be, knowing there's a patient in the next room wishing the doctor would hurry up? Your appointment with a psychiatrist means a structured amount of uninterrupted time is set aside for you and you alone.

I believe my general doctor is competent enough that if I had wanted drug therapy, he would have worked with me to find the right dosage level. But I knew what the source of my depression was. The loss of purpose, the rejection, and the crashing of my assumptions about life were all wound up inside me until I felt like I was going to explode. I was more than ready for a competent, probing listener.

If your doctor does not encourage you to see a therapist, it is still your prerogative to do so. If you don't know where to begin, the best thing to do would be to contact the nearest teaching hospital and request a list of names of psychotherapists who are well recommended and working in your area. Or, call the nearest university-affiliated psychiatric clinic.

3. We should recognize that seeking therapy is expensive. Some of us may be reluctant to get help at the prices charged, but when you consider what we spend to put new life into our cars and into our houses, it is not out of line to invest in ourselves as valuable people.

Some of us, though, simply don't have the money. I could not afford psychiatric help during my first two depressions, nor can I afford it now; so I understand the dilemma. At the time I saw a psychiatrist, we had a medical insurance policy that covered one-half of the cost. Different policies have different benefits to cover the treatment of depression.

If you can't afford to see a therapist and you don't have an insurance policy to cover treatment, look for a helping facility that offers counseling services. Begin treatment with a mental health professional—someone trained in counseling. If the counselor is competent, he should be able to tell if he can help you. If he can't, then it's a part of his job to know when and *where* to refer you. Counseling services such as those provided by churches charge less—

sometimes there is no cost—than psychiatric help. Look for churches and other helping agencies which have counselors on their staff.

The important thing is that if you fit one of the categories at the beginning of this chapter, you need outside help. Talk to someone competent in mental health. Don't try to make the determination yourself as to what kind of help you need. Go to someone who can make an appropriate diagnosis about depression and who will guide you wisely.

4. We are reluctant to seek professional help because we are Christians. In the Christian communities that I've been a part of, going to a psychiatrist or therapist has been looked down upon. As the pastor's wife of one of my relatives said to him, "You can either turn your problems over to the Lord, or you can see a psychiatrist." The two could simply never go together.

I didn't tell anybody I had made an appointment to see a psychiatrist. One of the reasons I didn't was because I was emotionally unable to handle their comments. On many occasions through our struggles, I had been hurt by the lack of regard other Christians had for our feelings. I was tired of Christians making light of my pain, and I wasn't going to give them another chance by telling them I was going to a psychiatrist.

Another reason I didn't tell was that I was afraid my admitting I needed help would prevent my getting to speak on prayer. I've written two books on prayer, and I like to speak on the subject; but I knew the question would be, why couldn't I just pray my way out of depression? (And I was right. I have been asked that question since I have started talking about my struggle with depression.)

But, speaking engagements or not, life was miserable and I wanted to feel better; so I kept my appointment with the psychiatrist. And I'll always be glad I did. During the first session, I wept through the entire hour. After I told Dr. Dubriwny what I had been through, he said, "You have reason to be depressed." Ah, here was my day in court!

The evidence was examined by a competent judge, and his verdict was, "Not guilty." So many had inferred that if I had had enough faith, if I had been strong enough as a Christian, then I would have had no reason to be depressed. Now, here was someone competent and knowledgeable, who could appreciate our ideals and our efforts in life and see why I had experienced such deep disappointment.

I also liked the release of talking out my hurts. I liked the dependability of knowing I had a set time to talk to the psychiatrist. What ever happened in between visits, I could somehow manage, just knowing that I would be seeing Dr. Dubriwny at our appointed time. He helped me see alternatives. As we talked about the consequences of the alternatives, he helped me see what I could and could not handle. It took me only four visits to be on my own again; but I'll always be glad I sought help.

Christian psychiatrists Minirth and Meier say that obtaining and applying good quality psychotherapy is synonymous with discipleship. "God sanctifies many people (brings them toward Christlikeness in their attitudes and behavior) through confrontation by loving and insightful friends, pastors, counselors—and even psychiatrists sometimes. Don't ever be ashamed to get counseling when going through life's stresses."[1]

Minirth and Meier were referring to Christian psychotherapy, but I think that applies to non-Christian psychotherapy, too, if the therapist respects your beliefs and values. Remember the therapist is trained to draw you out, to see your problems, and to help you clarify the issues. As long as he or she will allow you to talk about your spiritual side as well as your emotional and mental difficulties, you can benefit. Do not spend your time and money, however, with a therapist who will not respect your values.

One woman whose taped testimony I listened to spent twelve months with a therapist who would not let her mention anything spiritual! The minute he told her she couldn't talk about anything spiritual, she should have started looking for another therapist. We can't cut ourselves up into spiritual and mental and emotional selves as if one doesn't affect the other. We need to seek help from a competent therapist, who will let us be ourselves and express all of our values.

In addition to the stigma associated with Christians seeking psychological help, another problem that bothers some Christians is taking antidepressants or undergoing electroconvulsive therapy. There are times when depression can be fought without those helps, as we've already talked about in this book. Both my doctor and my psychiatrist offered to prescribe antidepressants for me, but I refused. I knew *why* I was hurting. My chronic depression was spiritually related, and I knew it was going to take some spiritual surgery and intense warfare to get well.

But suppose a person doesn't know why she is depressed; or suppose by the time she seeks help, she has lost a dangerous amount of weight; or suppose she is psychotic (breaking with reality), or intensely suicidal. People like this need immediate help. They need to be physically better before they can begin to tackle the emotional or spiritual side of their depressions. In older people, especially, appetite loss can have a truly dangerous significance. For the nutritional deficits resulting from weight loss during depression may literally be life threatening, as in the case of an elderly person.

> Malnutrition, and the bodily dehydration that results from it can lead to an irreversible process. If a certain physiological point-of-no-return is passed, the older person simply loses the ability to absorb and utilize the life-giving energy that is in our food—and the ability to absorb that energy doesn't return. The individual may begin eating again; but the food passes through the body without being taken up and used; and he or she therefore receives no nourishment. Once this process has been set into motion, the patient will ultimately die—of what hospital personnel call "the dwindles."[2]

In some cases, antidepressants or ECT may be necessary but there are Christians who still would be against either.

> They would say it is unspiritual to rely on medications at all since we should rely totally on the Lord. A century ago, a number of Christians thought it was a sin to wear glasses—or "devil eyes," as they called them. Their reasoning was, "If God wanted you to be able to see, He would have given you good vision." Even after penicillin was discovered, many Christians died of pneumonia because they wanted to trust God alone and not medication.[3]

Our attitude should be, "Thank God we have psychotherapy, antidepressants, and ECT." Depression is a very old disease. Many people through the years have suffered greatly because there was no help available. No person in this day and age needs to be depressed because it isn't treatable. There is lots of help available, and current research indicates that there will be even more help available in the years to come.

5. Even when we seek outside help with our depression, the route to recovery is still going to depend a lot on our *will.* In a lay witness mission, I talked about my difficulty with depression. Afterward, a woman said to me, "I've been depressed for seven years." There is no reason, with the kinds of help available today, for a person to be depressed that long unless she wants to be. If we want to, we can keep our depression and nobody in the world can take it from us. Our recovery is related to our will. Will we admit to having a problem? Do we want to get well? Doctors, counselors, and psychiatrists are available to help us, but they don't seek us out. We have to make the appointment. We have to go to them.

Therapists can help us through psychotherapy, antidepressants, and electroconvulsive therapy; but none of these things will work without our cooperation. A counselor can't make us talk. He can't be there each day to make us take a pill. He can prescribe ECT, but he cannot administer it against our will. Our will is very much a key to getting well, even when we seek outside help.

Seeking help and staying with it are hard acts for a depressed person. Our tendencies to withdraw, to think no one cares, to think a doctor couldn't really help us if we contacted him—all work against our recovery. We've got to make the effort and stick with the treatment.

The route each of us takes to get well may be different; but the important thing is that we've chosen a route. We want to get well. So, if you are hesitating to get outside help, the question you may need to ask yourself is the question Jesus asked the lame man by the pool of Bethesda (John 5:1-8). The lame man had been sick for thirty-eight years. When Jesus saw him, knowing the man had been sick for such a long time, he asked him, "Do you want to get well?"

[1]Minirth and Meier, *op. cit.*, p. 98.
[2]Scarf, *op. cit.*, p. 492.
[3]Minirth and Meier, *op. cit.*, p. 162.

ELEVEN

GETTING OVER DEPRESSION REQUIRES A CHANGE IN THINKING

In order to get over depression and stay free from it, I intuitively knew I was going to have to do some inner work in addition to seeking psychiatric help. (Here's one of those instances when being a woman is really helpful.) My perception was distorted. My thinking would have to be corrected if I were going to get well and stay well.

When I intensified my research on the subject of depression, I found that I had been right about the needed inner work. Many sources indicated that a change in thinking patterns is necessary to get over depression and stay over it. One Christian leader calls the work necessary to change thinking patterns: *spiritual* therapy. Another Christian leader calls it *prayer* therapy. Leaders in psychiatric research call it *cognitive* therapy. All three therapies insist that depression arises from erroneous thinking. Not only must the erroneous thinking cease, but new thoughts must replace the wrong ones.

SPIRITUAL THERAPY

Tim LaHaye, prominent Christian author, purports spiritual therapy in his best-selling book, *How to Win Over Depres-*

sion. He talks about the brain's two main sections—the conscious and the subconscious. Our present likes, dislikes, feelings, and reactions are engraved on our subconscious. They were probably engraved there during the impressionable days of our childhood and youth. Our experiences recorded impressions on our subconscious. These recorded impressions cause us to respond in certain ways to situations we face later in life. LaHaye says we are influenced more by our subconscious than by our conscious; and our subconscious is influenced by our imagination.

LaHaye compares our mind to a movie screen. Whatever our imagination flashes on the screen of our subconscious mind, dictates what we will do.

> Whatever you place on the screen of your subconscious mind will govern your activities. . . . Your imaginative self-image determines how you feel, and, as a result, how you work and act. The subconscious mind functions inexorably toward the fulfillment of whatever image you flash on the screen. . . .[1]

According to LaHaye, depressed people create negative, self-pitying pictures on the screen of their subconscious mind, inevitably making them feel depressed. By creating new images, they can gradually modify their feelings and their behavior. An individual can control his mind, feelings, and actions by projecting only beneficial images on the imagination of his mind. LaHaye calls this projection of what is beneficial on our mind screen, spiritual therapy.

COGNITIVE THERAPY

Dr. Aaron T. Beck of the School of Medicine of the University of Pennsylvania developed a method of treating depressive patients called "cognitive therapy." The basic premise of cognitive therapy is that our thoughts govern our moods. Self-defeating thoughts initiate bad moods. The way we look at things—our perceptions, our mental attitudes, and our beliefs—govern the way we feel.

In developing this therapy, Dr. Beck noticed that his patients were having unreported, self-critical thoughts running parallel to what they were saying out loud to him. What the patient said to Dr. Beck was not what the patient was saying to himself. The patient was experiencing two distinctive lines of thoughts running at the same time—one line was what the patient was saying out loud to Dr. Beck and the other line was unspoken, automatic thoughts. The patient was repeating the second line of thoughts to himself.

This second line of thoughts is an inner conversation with the self, usually quite critical in nature. Self accuses the self ("I'm no good," or, "I'm a complete failure"). The accusations are negative and they tend to distort reality. The accusations occur in a kind of mental shorthand with no logical sequence.

This second line of thoughts is dominated by a pervasive negativity. The world is perceived as dark and gloomy. Hopelessness permeates the thought patterns. With each negative, inner dialogue, depressive feelings and apathy increase.

This kind of inner thinking causes emotional turmoil, and it nearly always contains gross distortions. The thoughts appear valid, but many of them are irrational or just plain wrong. This twisted thinking is what cognitive therapists believe causes depression.

Dr. Beck discovered that people could be taught to identify and stop negative thoughts prior to experiencing the emotions that come from them; hence the development of cognitive therapy.

In a sense, cognitive therapy could be called thought therapy. A cognitive therapist challenges the depressed person to listen to her own negative thoughts. The therapist trains her to identify her inner saboteurs and silence them. This kind of therapy is very effective. Results come quickly, usually within a few weeks.

> ... Actually, cognitive therapy is the first form of psychotherapy which has been proven to be more effective than antidepressant drug therapy through rigorous scientific research under the critical scrutiny of the academic community. This therapy is unique in having professional evaluation and validation at the highest academic levels. It is *not* just another self-help fad but a major development that has become an important part of the mainstream of modern psychiatric research and practice. . . .[2]

A cognitive therapist helps the depressed person identify her negative ideas, images, and beliefs, then critically evaluate them and talk back to them. Dr. Beck has trained many counselors to use cognitive therapy with their patients. One person Dr. Beck has trained is Dr. David Burns. Dr. Burns has written a self-help manual for the depressed person to work herself free from depression and to stay free. In his book, *Feeling Good: The New Mood Therapy*, Dr. Burns offers a systematic approach that includes lots of self-help exercises to get over depression. He offers simple, concrete methods that can be applied on a daily basis. The book includes a test for determining whether you are depressed and how depressed you are. The test can be retaken at various points as you work through the exercises to see if you are making progress in getting over your depression.

PRAYER THERAPY

I was not aware of either LaHaye's spiritual therapy or Beck's cognitive therapy when I was trying to get over depression once and for all. But I was familiar with prayer therapy as outlined by Dr. William R. Parker and Elaine St.

Johns in *Prayer Can Change Your Life.* According to prayer therapy, depression is a symptom of something wrong in the inner kingdom. When we tackle what's wrong inwardly, supernatural help will come and help us get over being depressed.

We can correct what is wrong in the inner kingdom through prayer therapy. Prayer therapy involves surrender and affirmation. In surrender (or release, as I like to call it), we give God all the rubbish that is within us. We give God our fears, our guilt, our anger, our grief, our broken dreams, and our faulty assumptions. This concept of giving God something ugly may be hard for some of us to accept. We usually think of giving God something beautiful like a life or a special talent, and so forth. But the Bible says, "Casting all your care upon him; for he careth for you" (1 Peter 5:7).

It's very important, once this release of the rubbish has been accomplished, that we not quit praying. Our surrender creates a void within us. We must make certain that the void does not fill up again with the same rubbish we released. We must fill the void with positive, affirmative praying.

In affirmative praying, we put helpful, creative thoughts into that void. We affirm ourselves free of the rubbish we released, and we affirm the kind of person we want to be or the kind of things we want to replace the rubbish.

In my case, it meant renewing my belief in God having a purpose for us. I had mistakenly concluded that because I did not see a reasonable purpose in operation, there *was* no purpose. Tagged onto the loss of purpose was grief still left over from leaving the Bible training center and hurt over the disregard of our feelings by other Christians. Hopelessness about seeing any way out of our situation permeated my thinking. The hopelessness, the hurt, the grief, and the lack of belief in God's purpose—all had to go if I were to get well.

In releasing, I prayed, "Lord, I give you my hurts and my grief and my despair. I forgive the people whom I believed hurt me. I give you the past. I release it to you."

In affirmation, I prayed, "Today, Lord, I see myself as being free of depression and free of hurt. I see myself as feeling good about life again. I see you as smiling in approval of me because I remained faithful without understanding what was happening. I affirm my trust in you. I believe you have a purpose behind all that has happened. I'm hopeful about the future."

Changing our thinking through prayer, using surrender and affirmation, is not a one-time prayer experience. Changing our thinking, bringing it in accord with God's will, is a tenacious struggle. The first morning I prayed this way, the effects of it lasted about one hour. Then I was back wallowing in self-pity and hurt. The next morning, I prayed again in the same way. This time, the effect lasted a little longer.

Eventually, through surrender and affirmation, the day came when I was free of the trappings of the inner self, and I believed once again in the purpose of God. Incidentally, the evidence of purpose in our lives isn't any clearer now than when I was depressed. Due to the declining economy and the nature of the work, the life of an executive recruiter has been filled with lots of ups and downs. Bob and I continually have had to fight anxiety and insecurity. Coupled with this is our ongoing desire to serve the Lord. Through it all, Bob has tried to walk through doors in which he could serve God in a vocation, only to have the doors closed. So if I started judging our life by the evidence even now, I'd probably get depressed again! I don't make a judgment on the visible evidence; rather I choose to live and operate in the belief that God has a purpose for us. I believe our lives are counting for something. Believing that enables me to live free of depression and gives me the ability to cope with the confusion of our lives.

YOU'RE IN CHARGE

Whether it's spiritual therapy, cognitive therapy, or prayer therapy, there are some similar truths running through all three that we need to understand.

1. Thinking and depression are related. Either our erroneous thinking led to depression, or our thinking was distorted by the nature of the illness.

2. We must do something about our thinking in order to get over being depressed. An act of the will is needed. God can produce a change within us, but we must be willing to surrender our distorted thoughts.

3. Our erroneous thinking must be replaced by correct thinking. Our negative thinking must be replaced by positive thinking.

The importance of keeping one's mind clear of negative and harmful thoughts and replacing them with good, wholesome ideas is not a new concept. The New Testament is very clear about this.

Jesus warned us about protecting our inner self in a very strange parable that he told. He told about an evil spirit leaving a person and traveling over dry country, looking for a place to rest. If the evil spirit can't find a resting place, it says to itself, "I will go back to my house." The evil spirit goes back and finds the house he left clean and all fixed up. Then he goes out and brings home seven other spirits even worse than itself to live with him. Then the person who swept his house clean is in worse shape than he was at the beginning (Luke 11:24-26; Matthew 12:43-45).

If we think of our inner self as the house in Jesus' parable, the evil spirit represents our erroneous thoughts. We have to sweep our house clean to clear out those erroneous thoughts. But sweeping alone is not enough because those thoughts will return and bring more back with them! Hence, we need positive images, correct thinking, and affirming prayer to fill the vacuum created by sweeping the erroneous thoughts away.

Paul, too, teaches the importance of control over the inner self. In Colossians 3:2, he says, "Set your mind on the things above, not on the things that are on earth" (NASB). A certain mindset is required. In chapter 3, Paul lists some of the things that are to be put aside: immorality, impurity, passion, evil desire, greed, anger, wrath, malice, slander, and abusive speech (see Colossians 3:5, 8). Then he tells us what to put in their place: "Put on a heart of compassion, kindness, humility, gentleness and patience; bearing with one another, and forgiving each other ... *put on* love.... And let the peace of Christ rule in your hearts. ... Let the word of Christ richly dwell within you ... " (from Colossians 3:12-16, NASB). Paul's admonition to "put aside" and to "put on" are similar to the surrender and affirmation of prayer therapy.

At first glance, we may think Paul's words apply only to our thoughts and actions toward other people; but his words also speak of the way we treat ourselves. Aren't we guilty of slander against the self when we constantly put ourselves down? What about abusive speech such as, "How could I be so stupid?" or, "I never do anything right"? What about anger turned inward? Shouldn't we be compassionate, kind, and gentle toward ourselves as well as toward others?

How can we develop this mindset that Paul talks about? How can we let the peace of Christ rule in our hearts? How can we keep our inner house swept clean of evil thoughts?

We must become caretakers of our inner self. We must recognize the destructive force of our thinking, work diligently to get rid of erroneous thinking, and learn to keep our mind filled with positive, correct thinking.

One way to do this is to have a regular daily quiet time in which we consistently release the rubbish and spend time filling the remaining void with good things. Some of you may be thinking, "But, Brenda, you had a daily quiet time and that didn't keep you from getting depressed." No, it didn't, because I was not cognizant of what was happening. All of those devotional times I had weren't without meaning; but, in themselves, they were not a guarantee against depression. They were not insurance against depression because those phantom, automatic thoughts were running concurrently, and they were taking their toll.

Now that I understand depression and realize my vulnerability, I guard my inner self. I use my daily quiet time to assess my thoughts, attempting to correct wrong thinking and to eradicate harmful thinking. I'm also aware that positive, good thoughts must replace what I've eradicated. The replacement is made by affirmative praying and reading appropriate devotional material.

The Bible says, "Watch over your heart with all diligence, for from it flow the springs of life" (Proverbs 4:23, NASB). Diligently we must stand guard against wrong thinking, keeping it from making itself at home in our hearts. If we don't, self-defeating thinking will rob us of the joy of life and keep us from wanting to live.

If you are having a skeptical reaction to this chapter, you may be thinking, "I don't have any self-deprecating inner thoughts," or, "My thinking couldn't be distorted." Distorted thinking patterns run through our minds automatically without the slightest effort on our part to put them there. They come in and they make themselves at home. We become so comfortable with them we don't even know they are there.

Try listening to see. Ask the Holy Spirit to reveal them to you. Every time you feel depressed about something, try to identify a corresponding negative thought you had just prior to and during the depression. Or, when you are telling someone about your depression, start listening for a second conversation going on in your head. Once you've begun to hear these automatic thoughts, keep a note pad handy. Jot them down as they come. You might be surprised at what they say, and they may give you a clue as to why you are prone to depression.

I had always considered myself a positive person, but inwardly another thought system was being built. The self-pity and the cost-counting that I did during my struggle with depression fueled this inner thought system. The resulting fire raged so that my moods were affected in a destructive way. I became clinically depressed.

When I went to work on this inner thought system, I tackled the obvious distortions first—like not believing in a purpose for our lives. As I got well, I discovered other thought patterns that were wrong. They had been within for years, operating automatically, taking their toll on my zest for life. As I continue to work to eradicate them, I thank God for the awareness and subsequent freedom that has come.

There's a lot of disagreement in psychiatric circles about treating depression. Some experts say antidepressants are the only way; others say psychotherapy; and others say cognitive therapy. In these three chapters on getting over depression, I've tried to show what kind of help is available—emphasizing that there is not just one way out. In my opinion, they all have something to offer. But I'm especially thankful for the awareness of what I was doing to my inner self by the way I was thinking. Being a diligent caretaker of my inner self has set me free to enjoy life more fully.

[1]LaHaye, *op. cit.*, p. 127.
[2]Burns, *op. cit.*, p. 23.

TWELVE
HOW TO STAY FREE OF DEPRESSION

There is a euphoria that comes with getting over depression. It feels so good to be out of the pit of depression. The blues have vanished, and you just know that life will never get you down again. And it may not, for the depressive who experiences a one-time devastating loss—such as a woman who bogs down in her grief over her husband's death. After she works her way through it and finds a meaningful life, she may never have another problem with depression.

For others of us, those with recurring bouts of depression, the indication is that we have started to meet the changes of life with depressive reactions. We need a healthier response. We can't change life, but we can change the way we respond to it.

In light of our nature as women and in light of the nature of depression, there are key areas that must be given attention if we are to live free of depression. These key areas revolve around friendships, self-acceptance, feelings, unfinished business, and purpose. If we are willing to admit we need a healthier approach to life and if we are willing to work on these key areas, we can meet change with resiliency and courage rather than by becoming depressed.

DEVELOPING FRIENDS

Considering that unexpressed feelings lead to depression and that talking is a major part of getting well, it stands to reason that to stay free of depression, we need to talk on a regular basis. Women are sensitive; we see and observe a lot. And with our verbal skills, we need to express ourselves. For this, we need friends, and we particularly need women friends.

Men have buddies. With their nature as "do-ers," they do things with other men. They bowl, they fish, they hunt, and they work on old cars together. But when a man has an intimate friend, it is usually his wife. To her, he tells his innermost secrets and confidences.

A woman may have a friend in her husband, but she also needs female friends. A woman needs to share her intimate feelings and her interest in people and people's reactions. When women talk, they want an understanding listener. We want to tap that I-know-how-you-feel response. With our special sensitivity, we can tell when our listener is really sympathetic. A woman will have feelings she wants to share that her husband just cannot be sympathetic with. It is not that he is cruel or inconsiderate; he just can't give to his wife that I-know-how-you-feel response on many of the things she wants to talk about.

Or, with our eye for details, we may want to share more than he cares to hear. Many women soon get tuned out by their husbands or other male listeners when they insist on including too many details. If a woman wants to share all the details that are important to her, she usually needs a female listener. If a woman is seeing friends on a regular basis so that she is expressing her feelings, then unexpressed feelings are not going to pile up to the point of causing depression.

(A woman's conversations with her friends are *not* to take the place of conversation with her husband. A woman shouldn't be running to her friends with things she should be telling her husband. That would seriously harm the marriage relationship. A woman needs intimate sharing both with her husband and with her friends.)

In addition to finding a kindred spirit in other women, another reason we need female friends is because we are nurturers by nature. Because people are so important to us, we spend our lives caring for people around us. We make life better for our husbands, our children, and our bosses—but who looks after us? Through friendships, women look after each other. We show kindness and consideration for each other. We bring special touches of concern to the lives of our friends. We see the tired look of our friend with three preschoolers and say, "Let me watch the children this afternoon, so you can get a good nap." We see the tensed look of the female friend at the next desk and say, "Lunch is on me today." Without these touches of concern, a woman who is constantly giving to others begins to think nobody cares, providing fertile ground for depression.

Needing friends to look after us and to talk with is such a simple thing to understand. It's so basic that it seems as though the need for friends wouldn't have to be stated in a book directed toward Christian women. Yet it does, because developing and sustaining friendships is not easy in today's world. Here are some reasons why:

1. Our present society is not conducive to building and sustaining enduring friendships. Friendships take time. When women entered the marketplace in increasing numbers, both the women who went to work and those who stayed home were hurt. While both groups felt that nothing would change between them, things did change. It's a simple matter of arithmetic. Forty hours of time subtracted from one woman's week is a hunk of time. The woman who stayed home is reluctant to call her working friend when she is not at work; she realizes all the responsibilities that must be crammed into her working friend's at-home

hours. She is especially reluctant to call if her working friend has a husband and children. She doesn't want to take time away from them.

The woman who goes to work follows a tight schedule. When is there time for a leisurely cup of coffee with a friend? When is there time to be with "the girls"? Some women are fortunate to work in a kind of place where friendships with other women are possible. They simply left their "at-home" friends and replaced them with "at-work" friends. Other women in the working force are not so fortunate. Instead of finding friends, they found a new set of standards. In the competitive world of work, many women found themselves competitors instead of friends. A willingness to trust and to share one's innermost thoughts and feelings—so important to good friendships—can't often thrive in the harsh business world. As women become masculinized in their way of thinking in the competitive career climbing atmosphere, they learn that it is best not to reveal too much emotion or feeling. And besides, if a woman takes time to talk about her feelings or encourages someone else to talk, how is she going to get her job done? Meeting deadlines and maintaining quotas doesn't allow time for intimate sharing.

2. The mobile nature of our society makes it difficult to maintain friendships. We make a close friend and then we find we have to move, or she has to move. Often we are forced to live away from our extended families where female comaraderie was provided within the family—mother and daughter or sister and sister. We cannot have intimate day-by-day sharing and checking in with our mothers and sisters when we are living five hundred miles from them.

3. Our individualistic culture makes it hard to maintain friendships. Our culture emphasizes being strong and independent. This kind of emphasis makes it hard to admit we need others. We think we should be able to take care of our concerns by ourselves. We shouldn't need anybody else. If we do, it is a sign of weakness.

Sometimes, there is a similar emphasis in Christian circles: that if we are strong Christians, competent at prayer and Bible study, we should not need anybody else. Mark says that Jesus called the twelve apostles for two reasons: (1) to be with him, and (2) to send them out with a message and with power (Mark 3:14, 15). Jesus would need steady and consistent companions on the way to the cross. The crowds would come and go, but these twelve would be with him all the time.

God made us with a need for companionship and fellowship. He can use our friends as he uses prayer and Bible study to reach us and to communicate with us. It is not a weakness to need other people.

These three reasons are the major hurdles against forming and keeping friendships, but they are not the only reasons. Some of the hurdles are within us. We may be part of the problem. Our depressive way of thinking may be keeping us from enjoying the benefits of friends.

The woman prone to depression may want a friend to talk with and yet not want to make the effort. We want the other person to reach out to us. We want the other person to see our need and to know what is troubling us. We even send out signals—downcast eyes or a pained expression that say, "I'm hurting"—in the hopes someone will come to our aid without our having to do anything.

The signal that is so clear to us may not be noticeable to the person we are trying to attract. What may look like a flashing red light to us might not mean anything to the other person. That person we are trying to attract is busy with her own life and pursuits and even her own hurts. We can't count on others to read our mind. If we are going to live free of depression, we are going to have to stop leaning on our signals and speak up. There's no better way to begin than with these words: "I need your help."

The woman prone to depression may also want a perfect friend to tell her problems to. She had a friend "two moves back" who was ideal. Her friend shared her interests; she was a good listener, and she could almost read her thoughts. Nobody since can replace her. Maybe nobody can, but that doesn't mean valuable relationships can't be formed with different kinds of people.

The woman prone to depression may have been betrayed or hurt by a close friend once. At the time, she vowed, "I'll never get that close to another person again." So she holds off making friends, unwilling to trust again.

Like a spoiled child, the depressive's attitude is, "If I can't have friends the way I want them, then I won't have any friends at all." This everything or nothing kind of attitude is one of the unrealistic expectations depressives have about life and people. To have friends, we need to lessen our expectations.

We also need to develop more than one friend. It's *friends* we need. It's unrealistic to expect one person to always be available to listen to what we have to say. We might lose the one friend we have if we continue to unload all of our concerns on her. We might need to match the right trouble with the right friend. Some friends can listen to one thing but not another.

If you want to make friends, the best advice is found in Proverbs 18:24: "A man that hath friends must shew himself friendly." Ask yourself, what is friendly? How do I want someone to respond to me? Take your answers as guidelines for how to act to gain friends. Find a small group of Christian women to commit yourself to. Look for a group that is honest, nonjudgmental, and confidential. Don't join a group that has simplistic answers to all of life's problems. A group strong in listening and in caring is what a woman prone to depression needs.

A woman's Sunday school class, prayer group, or Bible study group offers precious sharing and fellowship. By *committing* yourself to the group, the members will get to know you and you them. Don't go one time and then pout because no one paid any attention to you. Friendship is a two-way street, and it takes time and commitment.

Friendships with other women are worth the time and commitment because of the nurturing support and the quality of listening we can receive. Maintaining friendships with other women should be high on the priority list of both working and nonworking women because it is vital to their mental health.

ACCEPTING MYSELF AS THE PERSON I AM

Because depression is a self-deprecating illness, a healthy sense of self-worth is needed to stay free of it. For me, developing a healthy sense of self-worth involved three areas: (1) accepting myself as the sinner I am, (2) loving myself as the person I am, and (3) accepting myself as the woman I am.

The first two may sound contradictory. How could I grow in realization of myself as a sinner and at the same time grow in regard for myself? Acknowledging our sinful nature and loving ourselves are both biblical truths that I had only partially applied to my life.

The Bible says, "For all have sinned and come short of the glory of God" (Romans 3:23). I could admit to being part of that "all," if we wanted to talk in terms of past tense. It was the future tense that I couldn't admit to.

There's always been within me an earnest desire to do everything right. I was a conscientious student of the Bible, an ardent pray-er, and an active church member. I put into practice whatever I was convinced was the truth. An A+ would not have been too high of a grade for the *effort* I put into living the Christian life. (This doesn't mean the results were any better or any worse than anybody else's life; it does mean that I tried very hard.) Subconsciously, I felt that if I kept reading, studying, and praying, then the day would come when I would do everything right. I would hold the key for not making any mistakes.

Depression blew that! I had tried so hard, and still my life fell apart. With the diagnosis of clinical depression, I had to admit that I do get angry, I do get hurt, and there is a limit to what I can handle.

Furthermore, I began to see that there was no guarantee against future frailty. If A+ effort could not guarantee perfection, then what could? I had to accept myself as a person who makes mistakes.

Life is a whole lot easier now. All that energy tied up in the frenzy to do right is now given over to enjoyment of life. I can do more things and enjoy them more because they don't have to be done exactly right.

In addition to accepting myself as a sinner, I also had to come to love myself. When Jesus commanded us to love God and to love our neighbor, he said to love our neighbor as we love ourselves (Mark 12:30, 31). A healthy relationship with our neighbors requires loving ourselves.

Rejection was one of the causes of my depression. The way I viewed our situation, everybody was rejecting us. It was *their* fault. One evening in a small group study, my husband gave us a questionnaire to determine our degree of self-acceptance. The results surprised me.

Here is the little test I took, in case you might like to try it. Answer the questions the way you genuinely feel.

True___ False___ 1. I received from my parents about all the love I needed.

True___ False___ 2. I am no more self-conscious than the average person.

True___ False___ 3. I seldom feel terribly critical of people.

True___ False___ 4. I have about as many friends as I would like.

True___ False___ 5. It doesn't bother me much when people I know do something stupid.

True___ False___ 6. I think I have gotten about as much as I deserve from life.

True___ False___ 7. I have not been bothered by many physical or emotional symptoms.

True___ False___ 8. I tend to trust most people without too much difficulty.
True___ False___ 9. Politicians are about as honest as the average person.
True___ False___10. I am probably no more sensitive than most people.
True___ False___11. It seldom occurs to me that people might be laughing at me.
True___ False___12. Most people won't let you down in a pinch.[1]

Count the number of trues checked. Six trues is average. Anything above that indicates a good to high degree of self-acceptance. Any score *below six* suggests a weak self-image.

I scored below six. No wonder the rejection we experienced hurt so much. The rejection was added evidence to support my own low view of myself.

Self-esteem must be remedied from within. A healthy self-esteem cannot be based on our achievements. It cannot be based on the opinion of others, because their opinions will change. It cannot be based on physical attractiveness, because physical attractiveness can be lost or destroyed. A healthy sense of self-worth must come from within, from a person's own regard for self.

To remedy my low sense of self-worth, I prayed, "God, help me to love myself. Help me appreciate the person you've created. Help me to see that I have value just because I am. Help me to see that I can make a unique contribution to your kingdom."

Along with accepting ourselves as the sinners and as the persons we are, we need to accept ourselves as the women we are. Acceptance doesn't mean resignation; acceptance means awareness. Awareness of our nature gives us a handle on living with ourselves: In light of the way I am, how then do I respond to life?

For example, women find great meaning in relationships.

The main cause of depression for women is loss of relationships. Does that mean we should avoid relationships so that we can stay free of depression? No, for to do that would deny our womanliness. What we must do is to learn to handle our vulnerability.

How can we handle our vulnerability? We can believe there will be a life for us after the loss. We can develop interests that will help carry us through. We can grieve when the loss occurs, knowing the grieving process is healthy.

Many women will, at some point in their lives, have to live alone. Women, on the average, outlive men by seven to eight years. Some women whose identity has been solely in terms of their mates will think of the death of their mates as death for themselves. They think they can't survive if their husbands don't. Accepting ourselves as women says, "I'm not afraid to face the possibility of living alone. I will learn to be strong and gain useful skills so that when a relationship ends, I will survive. I will grieve, knowing it is a process that will end." This is a much healthier approach than burying the fear and refusing to acknowledge the loss.

In accepting ourselves as women, we need to accept ourselves as biological creatures. Changes within our bodies do affect our moods. We need to live in harmony with the way God made us instead of expecting ourselves to be superwomen and super Christians every day of our lives. The prayer life of Jesus shows us how very much we need to have time for spiritual replenishment if we are going to be constantly giving.

Women, as people-lovers who invest so much in their love bonds, are in a position of continually giving. This can be spiritually draining. Women need time in which to be refreshed. The days of premenstrual tension could be just that—a time for spiritual recharge and a time when we don't make so many demands on ourselves.

Practically speaking, that may mean taking an afternoon out on the couch and reading a good, inspirational book.

If you are employed, it may mean saving your money and letting your husband take the children out to eat while you enjoy an evening home alone. Let the days of premenstrual tension be days in which you are good to yourself. In this way, the biological rhythm of life can help you invest in your emotional bank on a regular basis.

As the women we are, and given our natures, we are not going to be free of being *vulnerable* to depression. But we can keep ourselves free from succumbing to it, by accepting and living with our nature rather than repressing our fears and ignoring our biology.

GETTING IN TOUCH WITH OUR FEELINGS

Depression thrives on unexpressed feelings. Catching on to what we are feeling and what triggers the feeling can be very valuable in learning to live free from depression.

We need to learn to recognize our feelings and identify them. There's no one way to do this. Here are a few suggestions for getting started:

Relax and don't try so hard. Just be yourself.

Start listening to the inner self.

Ask the Holy Spirit to help you recognize your feelings.

Read some good books on feelings. Learn the characteristics of particular feelings such as anger, grief, fear, guilt, and anxiety. The greater the awareness of what we are feeling, the greater our control.

Once we recognize our feelings, we need to learn appropriate ways to deal with them. We can't just start unleashing all of our newly recognized feelings on those we live with. There are appropriate ways to deal with feelings. Here are three suggestions:

1. *Give in to the feeling.* Although feelings of fear, anger, anxiety, and sadness are unpleasant, we should allow ourselves to experience them. It is not going to hurt to be anxious or sad for awhile. Letting ourselves experience feelings neutralizes them. Neutralizing them causes them

to disintegrate. Burying them preserves them.

For example, no one is going to live free of depressive feelings. When they come, allow yourself to be depressed. Take the afternoon off. Get a good night's sleep. Tomorrow the feelings may be all gone because you did not fight them. (A woman who has had a problem with depression may panic when depressive feelings return. She may think, "Oh, no, here I go again." But there is no reason for concern unless the depressive feelings persist for more than two weeks.)

Another example is mourning. When we mourn or express deep feelings of disappointment, the act in itself is healing. Perhaps this is the wisdom in the Beatitude, "Blessed are they that mourn: for they shall be comforted" (Matthew 5:4). The mourning process is a release, a healing that paves the way to recovery.

2. *Learn to articulate your feelings.* Suppose your husband often makes you angry. In the past, in trying to be a good wife, you kept your feelings to yourself and consequently you were often depressed. To live free of depression you are going to have to find a way to appropriately express your anger. Don't start unloading on him the minute he gets home from work. Some planning and forethought will make your expression of anger easier for him and for you. Say, "Dear, tonight when the children are in bed, I need to talk some things over with you." Emphasize your *need* to talk, not his actions that have made you angry. What you are wanting is a chance to express your feelings, not a chance to hurl accusations at him.

Sometimes it may help to give yourself an escape valve before you talk with him, venting some of your anger. Air your anger at your husband with a confidential friend before you present your case to your husband. This will neutralize a lot of the anger so you will be more rational when you talk with him. My husband says he can handle anything I have to say, as long as it isn't said with tears! I don't always succeed, but I try to get my crying done before I tell him how I feel.

3. *Engage in honest praying.* Many depressives hate mornings, when they experience a worsening of symptoms. My bad times were around four o'clock in the afternoon. I would get up in the morning, pray, and affirm God's love and purpose for me. But then little things would happen throughout the day that would trigger memories. All the hurt would roll back in, and the black, bleak sadness of depression would converge on me. I had to find a way to deal with those four o'clock blues if I was going to live free of depression.

The answer for me was honest praying. In our bathroom (the only room in the house with a lock on the door!) is a built-up step, just right for an altar. When the four o'clock blues hit, I would flee to the bathroom, close the door, and fall on that step. There I would let the tears flow and unleash my anger and hurt. "God, how could you do this to us? How could you hurt us when we tried so hard to serve you? How could you abandon us?" I would say everything I felt until the emotion was spent. Then something would click inside, and suddenly God didn't seem so far away. New strength would fill me, and I'd feel as if I could cope. I'd get up, wash my face, open the door, and go out to meet the world again, free of the feelings that drove me to pray.

Some Christians might question the "rightness" of honest praying; how could I talk to God like that? Honest praying opens the way for God to come in and do a work of grace in our hearts. Jesus' prayer life is filled with honesty as he expressed his feelings. In front of a group of people, as he was headed toward Jerusalem and the cross, he said, "Now is my soul troubled" (John 12:27). Alone, while his disciples slept nearby, Jesus prayed for an escape from the cross (see Mark 14:32-42; Matthew 26:36-46; Luke 22:39-46). On the cross, we hear Jesus' awful cry, "My God, my God, why hast thou forsaken me?" (Mark 15:34).

Each time, God ministered to Jesus. After Jesus prayed, "Now is my soul troubled," God gave him strength to go on to Jerusalem toward the cross. After his plea for escape in the Garden of Gethsemane, God strengthened Jesus in such a way that he calmly proceeded toward the cross. As the drama of Jesus' last hours unfolded, Jesus, more than Pilate, more than those who sought his arrest, appeared to be in control. After his cry of abandonment from the cross, fellowship between the Father and the Son was restored. Jesus died with a shout of triumph on his lips (John 19:30) and a prayer of restored fellowship, "Father, into thy hands I commend my spirit" (Luke 23:46).

When we cannot understand, when we cannot see how God could possibly be at work in our circumstances, then it is all right to pray, "My God, why have you forsaken me?"

Neutralizing our feelings by giving in to them, learning to articulate our feelings in an acceptable manner, and honest praying are three ways in which we can handle our feelings. There are other ways, but these three should give us something to start with as we learn to recognize our feelings in order to live free of depression.

WORKING ON UNFINISHED BUSINESS

Unfinished business provides breeding ground for growing depressive episodes. If we are going to live free of depression, then we are going to have to take care of the unfinished business in our lives.

Some unfinished business is hidden business. It is buried so deep that it would take professional counseling to eradicate it. If you suspect this may be part of your problem, you may want to seek professional counseling.

On the other hand, there is plenty of obvious unfinished business that we can take care of if we are willing to do the necessary work.

Unresolved guilt. Guilt, whether false or real, needs to

be resolved. As long as it isn't, it stands in the way of our fully experiencing the benefits of God's forgiveness.

Unforgiveness of parents or siblings. All persons are damaged, in some degree, by their environment; but that is no cause to blame our struggle with depression on our parents. They, and we, are usually doing our very best, however poor that may be. If a woman wants to live free of depression, she needs to learn to accept her parents and her brothers and sisters as people. It's all right for them to be the way they are; and it's all right for her to be the way she is.

Living as a little girl, afraid of being her own person. A woman may try hard to live by the standards of her parents instead of her own. For her, the separation so necessary for good mental health has not occurred so that she might enjoy her relationships with her parents as an adult with adults.

While we work to clear up unfinished business from the past, we also want to make sure we don't leave unfinished issues from the depression we are currently trying to get over. We get hurt easily when we are depressed. We misread what other people say and do. We feel slighted. The temptation is to overmagnify these hurts and file them away in our inner person. In the euphoria of getting over the physical symptoms, we think those filed-away feelings aren't going to matter. But they do. They can become breeding ground for future depressive episodes unless we work to eradicate them.

To make sure we clear up unfinished business from our current depression, we must be careful when we take antidepressants. With antidepressants, there's the temptation of wanting to think the cause of our depression is purely physical so that we will not have to do any inner work on ourselves. Antidepressant drugs relieve depressive symptoms, but they do not cure the causes.

Many grief experts feel that antidepressant drugs should not be used for persons going through normal grief and mourning, nor for persons who can fairly easily identify the loss that has triggered the depression. If the grief and unexpressed emotions are not worked through, they become "unfinished business" for precipitating another depressive episode later on. To live free of depression requires a willingness to work on the unfinished business in our lives.

LIVING WITH PURPOSE

The author of Hebrews writes about the "rest" of God. (See Hebrews 3:7—4:10.) For us today, the rest of God is synonymous with the peace of God. The peace of God comes to us when we trust and obey him. This trust and obedience is not a casual thing; it's the kind of thing we would stake our life on. It means we believe what God says is true. It means we believe that what God says he can do, he will do. When we obey accordingly, the peace of God enters our lives.

The peace of God eluded me when I stopped believing he had a purpose for Bob and me. No purpose meant no trust; and without trust, I was miserable.

The happiest times in my life were the times I completely trusted God. For me, to live a life free of depression meant living a life of trust. A life of trust did not change the earthly circumstances. The road of an executive recruiter has been a rough one in a spiraling-downward economy. Our livelihood is always uncertain; but I live in the trust that someday this is all going to make sense. This trust gives me a long-range handle on life, rather than letting my emotions ride up and down with our livelihood.

Much of what I have read on depression recommends goals for living; other material recommends adding structure to one's life. Both of these recommendations have merit. Women need goals; they need to think about what kind of women they want to be. When we make choices in line with the kind of woman we want to be, we are exerting some control over our lives instead of letting everyone else or everything else control us.

Short-range goals also help. They help us direct our living and provide structure for using our energy. Many women enjoy a job for this reason. The job gives structure to her responsibilities. She must arrange for a time to cook, a time to clean, a time to work, and a time to relax.

Goals and structure help us with the business of living, but both of these things may be operative and a woman still may miss the "rest" of God. She can become depressed if something happens to her structure or if she reaches her goal. "What do I do now?" she may ask. A healthier approach calls for a philosophy of life that is ongoing and independent of goals and structure. A woman needs a meaningful purpose for her life. Much of what a woman is responsible for could be described as humdrum. She needs a purpose for living that will make the humdrum significant.

Committing our life to God's Son, Jesus, can give significance to what we do. Commitment means that I believe what Jesus says to be true. Commitment means doing everything in our power to live like him. Commitment also means continuing to follow Jesus no matter what the circumstances are. When we do, we receive the rest of God.

William Barclay calls this rest of God, "the rest we dare not miss." We dare not because to be at peace with God is the greatest thing in the world. I know because I tried to live without it.

We must not be misled by the euphoria that follows depression and start making grandiose claims. The euphoria is a contrast in feelings between what it feels like to be out of the pit of depression and being in it. The euphoria is not a guarantee against future depressive reactions. If there is a guarantee, it comes in working hard to stay free. That means developing friends, accepting ourselves, getting in touch with our feelings, working hard on unfinished business, and living with purpose. These things are not easy to accomplish, but they do provide targets for developing a response to life that is not a depressive one.

[1]Cecil G. Osborne, *The Art of Learning to Love Yourself* (Grand Rapids, Mich.: Zondervan Publishing House, 1976), p. 154.

THIRTEEN
HOW TO GAIN FROM DEPRESSION

A lovely line in the last chapter of Job says, "So the Lord blessed the latter end of Job more than his beginning . . ." (Job 42:12a). That same line may be written about the conclusion of our own despair. Depression can be a valley of reconstruction, so that when we emerge, the rest of life can be better than it was before we were depressed.

I'm not trying to romanticize depression. If anything, I hope this book has shown how horrible depression is. Depression is not the kind of experience we would ever deliberately want to seek out. But once we have it, good things can come out of it—good, life-changing things that make life all the better for having had the experience. I saw this in everyone I talked with who acknowledged they had been depressed and had *really* gotten over it. Depression had been a turning point for them, so that now they face life with new freedom and new views. The new views were varied. Some gained a new view of life; others a new view of themselves or of other people. Most gained a new view of God.

NEW VIEW OF LIFE

At first, when our unrealistic expectations are challenged and shot down, we're so dismally disappointed that we think, "If this is life, who wants it?" In struggling with depression, our expectations have to be reviewed. In getting well, some of them have to be discarded. Maybe the discarding was long overdue. The search for grandiose dreams or the attempt to reach unrealistic goals or the clinging to falsely based beliefs needed reevaluation.

For example, the concept that I held about always having the regard of your fellow Christians if you were a conscientious Christian was an erroneous one. Jesus' actions and teachings were met with ridicule, with rejection, and with death from the religious leaders of his day. Friction or disagreement with other church people may be a sign that we are indeed being like Jesus. Being a strong Christian may attain the regard of one's fellow Christians, or it may not. I needed the courage to serve God either way. Depression helped me see that I was too dependent on what other Christians thought of me.

As Christians, it's so easy to create an artificial world out of unrealistic expectations. Stan Mooneyham said it well in one of his columns when he was president of World Vision International:

> This side of the Third World we have almost convinced ourselves that, for Christians, the going is not supposed to be rough; we're not supposed to become depressed, have marital problems, generation gaps, business failures, sorrows. Tragedy, we say, is something that happens to unbelievers, and if it does overtake the faithful, we presume it to be embarrassing evidence of a flawed faith. So we engage in the Big Cover-up, cloaking our humanity, our hurts, our failures—not under a mantle of love, but behind a curtain of deceit—because we cannot face the exposure of being honest and real.[1]

The loss that caused our depression may have taught us in a very vivid way that tragedies and perplexities happen to Christians. The Bible has never painted the picture of life any other way; it is our distortion of biblical truth that makes us think otherwise. It's time we come of age and realize that faith is not a guarantee of a way of life; rather it is a muscle to be exercised in the ongoing struggles of life.

A Christian woman can gain from depression if she learns to deal honestly with life. Depression can help her be honest about her own perplexities as well as share in the perplexities of others. She knows life brings surprises; she knows life is often unfair. She also knows she is vulnerable to being overcome by the harshness of life. This knowledge, though, is not shackling. Instead, it heightens her sensitivity of life, frees her to be herself, and makes her an active participant in life.

Roy W. Fairchild says, "Depression is often an inherent part of the process of first coming apart, then recovering new insight, and finally giving up old perspectives that no longer fit our life."[2] When we do, we'll find life after depression better than life before depression.

NEW VIEW OF SELF

A woman who really works through her depression and overcomes it emerges from the experience with precious new insights about herself. She has a greater self awareness and a firmer sense of "who I am." She feels a new strength and her fear of aloneness is diminished. She realizes she is a person of value, and she respects that.

This was so true in my own life that I felt like a female version of Lazarus. The Gospel writer John tells us about Lazarus, how he died, was buried, and how Jesus brought him back to life. At the grave site, Jesus reminds Lazarus' sister, Martha, that he, Jesus, is the resurrection and the life (John 11:25). That promise is true for the depressed who no longer want to live, as well as for those who actually die, as Lazarus did.

Just as surely as the grave clothes were wrapped around the lifeless body of Lazarus, my depression wrapped itself around me, choking out the pleasures of this life and the desire for any future.

In the process of getting well and staying well, I felt as though the grave clothes were slowly unwound and a new me emerged. I like the new me very much.

The new me expresses her feelings more freely. She tells her husband how she feels. This doesn't take anything away from her submissive role as a Christian woman. In fact, her husband likes her better this way.

The new me admits to having aggressive feelings, especially in the realm of the spiritual. She has more courage now about expressing those feelings; it's a matter of integrity. She's not always right, but at least she feels free to say what she believes.

The new me admits when she needs help. Rather than people liking her less because she admits her frailties, they seem to like her more. Who wants a friend who isn't human?

The new me knows that she is loved for herself. She does not have to be perfect to be loved.

The new me knows what a trap the subconscious can be. Consequently, she has a greater awareness and appreciation for spiritual warfare. She understands the subtlety of the enemy and realizes she'll always have a fight on her hands.

The new me knows it is all right to fail. Having everything go right in one's life doesn't necessarily indicate spiritual maturity. As one pastor said, "Jesus will not say on judgment day, 'Well done, thou good and *successful* servant.' He will say, 'Well done, thou good and *faithful* servant.' Being faithful is what counts."

These changes have been good for me. While I would

never choose to have been depressed, neither would I have wanted to live the rest of my life without learning these things about myself. I like the woman that depression set me free to be.

NEW VIEW OF OTHERS

Gaining from depression may include a new view of others. The woman who successfully works her way through depression may drop her one-dimensional view of life and start looking at those around her more objectively. When she does, she may get a new view of her husband, her children, her friends, or her co-workers.

One woman who was overly conscientious said, "In order to live free of depression, I had to come to grips with the fact that there would always be people who littered, who were late to church, and who would mow their yards on Sunday. I could not change them, but I could learn to live with them. I haven't relaxed my standards for myself, but I have stopped trying to force my standards on others. For me, that spells progress."

It was imperative that if I were to stay free of depression I was going to have to learn to live with other Christians. When I was in college I became disappointed in the behavior of some Christian leaders. That was my first experience of seeing how unkind and manipulative people could be in the name of Jesus. I rebelled against God for awhile because of my disappointment. Later, when God brought me back to him, I went to seminary where I met mature, responsible, and kind Christian leaders. The seminary experience was a renewing one. I "shelved" my college experience as a "one-time" lesson with the belief that it would not happen again. ("Shelving" is an example of unfinished business.)

Then years later through our experiences with a Christian university, with a Bible training center, and with a large church, I learned there were more Christians like some of those I had known in college. I despaired again of the behavior of Christians. Did we really belong to the same family of God? If I were going to follow Jesus, then I was going to have to find a way to live with them.

A conversation between Peter and Jesus gave me a handle on learning to live with other Christians. When Jesus indicated to Peter that he would suffer a martyr's death for the gospel's sake (John 21:18, 19), Peter wanted to know if John's life would end in the same way (John 21:20, 21). "Jesus answered him, 'If I want him to live until I come, what is that to you? Follow me!' " (John 21:22, TEV). In other words, Peter should be concerned about his own relationship to Jesus rather than another's. Each of us must be responsible for our own actions. Preoccupation with another believer's behavior will only detract from our commitment.

I had to stop dwelling on the behavior of other Christians. My preoccupation with their behavior didn't change or influence them in any way. I had to focus my attention on my own relationship with Jesus. This doesn't mean I condone everything other Christians do. Far from it, I speak out when I can, but I have stopped dwelling on the injustices.

All Christians are sinners living out a commitment to Jesus Christ. Because we follow Jesus, I can live and work with them. That doesn't mean I condone their behavior, but it does mean I can call them "brother" and "sister."

NEW VIEW OF GOD

For Christians, depression has a spiritual dimension. Getting over it and living free of it will naturally include gaining new spiritual insights or theological understandings. One of the more common gains is unconditional acceptance by God. Many are glad to learn through their depression that God accepts them just as they are.

> So, fundamentally, we manage depression by realizing that we belong to God, and that we do not have to do one thing in the world to be worthy. We are significant because we are who we are. We are valuable, not because we perform well; we are not dealing with good and bad. That is not the point. We are valuable because we are ourselves. God loves us! God loves us exactly as we are! Should that ever dawn on us, we may be depressed periodically, and we will sometimes experience sadness, but I am here to tell you that we will not be overcome by it![3]

One woman had God's love mixed up with her father's love. Her father had been extremely success-oriented. Whatever his children accomplished was not good enough; he always demanded more. This woman responded to God as she had been taught to respond to her earthly father. She kept on doing more and more to try to please God, only to wind up totally exhausted and depressed. Her recovery hinged upon her coming to distinguish God from her father.

Another woman had quite the opposite experience. Her view of God was of a good daddy who gave his favorite daughter what she wanted. Then when the events of life didn't go as she expected, she found out—as she puts it—that she did not have God wrapped around her little finger.

These are concepts of God that needed changing. Sometimes our theology can only be put right when it is challenged by the circumstances of life. But in evaluating our theology, in getting over depression, life becomes freer and our relationship with God is better because we know him more accurately.

Depression did not give me a new view of God; rather it made vivid a nebulous belief. I had always believed in the holding power of Jesus Christ. In my struggle with depression, I experienced it. Many were the times when I wanted to give up Christianity altogether. As I went to church and became upset, I would think, "I could get over being depressed if I just gave up church altogether." So, during times of contemplation, I could see myself not going to church again. In my mind I would picture the Christian activities I could eliminate from my life. Across the picture would come Jesus, dusty and bloody, carrying his cross, wearing his crown of thorns, experiencing the ultimate in rejection. With weary, sad eyes, he would say to me, "Brenda, I thought we were in this together." With those words and that look, I knew that I could never reject him. I love him far too much for that. I am a Christian today and will continue to be because of Jesus.

A new view of God, a new view of others, a new view of self, and a new view of life are all gains that can come from getting over depression. Leslie D. Weatherhead refers to these gains as "treasures of darkness."

> Like all men, I love and prefer the sunny uplands of experience, when health, happiness, and success abound, but I have learned far more about God, life, and myself in the darkness of fear and failure than I have ever learned in the sunshine. There are such things as the treasures of darkness. The darkness, thank God, passes. *But what one learns in the darkness, one possesses forever.*[4]

There is no pit of depression so deep that God cannot bring a gain out of it. It may take our admitting we have a problem, and it may take our asking someone (professional or nonprofessional) to walk out of it with us. Nevertheless, the possibility for gain is still there.

With life full of "cast-down" places, clinical depression can't always be avoided. Sometimes it catches us unaware as it did me. But women are great synthesizers of information. We can "take in" a subject, absorb it, and make appropriate application so that with God's help, even a devastating experience like depression can become life-enhancing. Whether it is life-enhancing will depend a lot upon our own attitude and our willingness to work. The question is: Do we *just* want to get over depression or do we want to gain from it? That soil of vulnerability that predisposes women to depression can also be soil for a thriving, abundant life. The possibility of one automatically includes the possibility of the other. Which will it be for you?

[1]Stan Mooneyham, *World Vision*, February, 1982, p. 23.
[2]Roy W. Fairchild, *op. cit.*, p. 77.
[3]Barry Bailey, *Living with Your Feelings* (Nashville, Tenn.: Abingdon Press, 1979), p. 53.
[4]Leslie D. Weatherhead, *Prescription for Anxiety* (Nashville, Tenn.: Abingdon Press, 1956), pp. 30, 31.

FOURTEEN

HELPING OTHERS GET OVER DEPRESSION

Perhaps you chose to read this book because you know a woman who is depressed, and you would like to help her. As her husband, friend, neighbor, Sunday school teacher, or sister, you are in a good position to help her. You can initiate contact. The mental health professional must wait for the depressed woman to make an appointment and come to his office. The professional is dependent upon regularly scheduled appointments; but those who love her as a friend or spouse are in a position to seek her out and to be available at irregular times. The seeking out and the availability will mean much to the depressed woman who's certain no one cares.

In your concern for her and in your desire to help, here are some guidelines to consider.

1. *Learn what you can about depression.* You have already taken the first step in helping by reading this book. You need to know that depression is an illness. You need to know its symptoms and its causes. This will help you to recognize the illness in her, and, at times, clarify with her what is happening. Knowing the causes will help you

see what triggered her depression. It's important, too, that you know the illness is self-lifting. This will help you in being patient with her and being hopeful about the outcome. Learning about the illness of depression will help you in relating to her and in your ability to walk through the illness with her.

2. *Encourage the depressed woman to talk about her feelings.* The depressed woman needs your listening presence. You do not need to talk or probe or offer advice in order to help her. She needs you to be with her and to listen to her. Many times, especially during my first depression, I longed for someone just to sit and "brood" with me. That may sound morbid, but I was baffled by the actions of God. I wanted someone to ponder his mysterious ways with me. Few people have the time or desire to "just be" with a depressed woman. If you do have time and are willing, you have a valuable gift to give to her. Your presence during a time of intense despondency shows your love and will help counteract the rejection she is feeling.

Don't expect a depressed woman to reach out for support. Confer it anyway. In this book, I have tried to get the depressed woman to realize her need for others. I have encouraged her to admit her need for help—an act that is going to be very hard for her to do. For some with a low sense of self-worth simply may not be able to reach out. You can help that woman by reaching out to her.

While she very much needs to talk, don't push. Let her know you're there and ready to listen when she is ready to talk. Encourage her to talk about her feelings. You may have to ask repeatedly until she is convinced of your genuine concern and believes she can trust you. Listening appropriately to a depressed person is not easy. Here are some guidelines.

(a) Do not interrupt with your own experiences. A woman revealing her inner troubles does so after much self-questioning and is in a highly emotional state. A rough interruption, even if it is well intended, may be enough to discourage her. This doesn't mean you should say nothing. You may wish to ask a question now and then to get her story clear in your mind. But if you intrude with your experiences in the middle of her story, she will think you are putting her down or are not taking her troubles seriously enough.

(b) Do not condemn. The very fact that a person is willing to confess her troubles means that she is clearly aware of the situation. To condemn is to pile guilt upon guilt until she'll stop talking about her inner troubles. There may come a time in your relationship when you can offer advice, but don't give it until you have listened to her often and gained her confidence.

(c) Do not be shocked. If you have repeatedly tried to get her to say what is bothering her and then you react in disbelief, she'll look upon your shock as condemnation. She'll clam up, and it will be difficult for anyone to get her to talk again about her inner troubles. Even the half-concealed indrawing of the breath when a woman says a rather startling thing may end the confidence.

(d) Do not betray a confidence. This is hard to keep; frankly, very few people can keep a confidence. Don't be tempted to tell another person, prefacing your remarks with, "Now I know you won't tell anybody, but . . ." or, "I am telling you in the greatest confidence," and then proceed to reveal what you were asked not to tell. A depressed woman needs the assurance that what she reveals will not be repeated.

Roy M. Fairchild says, "Hope is born when someone really *hears* us."[1] You can give a depressed woman hope by listening to her when that listening is not disruptive, not shocked, not condemning, but confidential. A good verse for those who want to help the depressed is James 1:19: "My dear brothers, take note of this: Everyone should be quick to listen, slow to speak and slow to become angry" (NIV).

3. *Try to understand how she feels.* A step beyond lis-

tening is trying to understand how the depressed woman feels. Women need to have their feelings validated and accepted. They do not seek solutions as much as understanding. Later on, perhaps, there may be a right moment to help her seek solutions; but when a woman is depressed, she wants first to be listened to.

Perhaps the reason a depressed woman succumbs to her lonely feelings and withdraws is that she thinks no one will understand. One dictionary definition of depression is sadness greater and more prolonged than warranted by any objective reason. Perhaps she senses the exaggeration of her complaint and doesn't seek anyone out, fearing she will be made fun of or belittled because of her concerns. This kind of loneliness—that there is no one who understands—is awful to experience.

> The most acute kind of loneliness is not caused by the absence of other persons. It is the aloneness that engulfs us when we are unable to sense that others are sharing, caring, supporting, or identifying with us in a time of great need.[2]

Because the complaint of the depressed woman does seem exaggerated to the nondepressed person, it is hard not to dismiss her concerns. Parents may be tempted to respond to female adolescent depression with denial: "What do you have to be depressed about? These are the best years of your life!" Such parents have forgotten how painful the transition from childhood to adulthood can be for many people.

Don't say to a depressed woman, "It's all in your head." Or, "I know plenty of women who would trade places with you." Or, "You've really got a lot to be thankful for." Or, "If you'll just turn this over to the Lord, your problems will be solved." There may be some truth in each of these statements, but your saying them *too soon* says you are not taking her problems seriously. The underlying message is, "I do not understand how you feel, and I do not care to try."

The healing of depression is a process. A woman who is hurting needs to be listened to and have her feelings validated as a part of the process. Don't try to bypass the process by giving trite responses to her pain. This will take a lot of self-restraint; but she wants and needs the camaraderie of understanding more than she needs solutions.

4. *Don't be overly cheerful.* "Like one who takes away a garment on a cold day, or like vinegar poured on soda, is one who sings songs to a heavy heart" (Proverbs 25:20, NIV). *Today's English Version* of the Bible puts it this way, "Singing to a person who is depressed is like taking off a person's clothes on a cold day or like rubbing salt in a wound."

If someone you cared about was cold, you wouldn't take his coat away. If someone you cared about was wounded, you wouldn't rub salt in his wound. If you care about someone who is depressed, then you won't be overly cheerful. A depressed person finds a loud, cheerful person irritating. Loud laughter and excessive hilarity grate on her nerves. Don't slap her on the back and say, "Praise the Lord!" or "Cheer up, things could be worse." Florence Littauer says, "The depressed person needs a loving, understanding mate, not a cheerleader."[3]

This doesn't mean you should succumb to her sadness, but it does mean that you should not view her situation frivolously. Be hopeful in a quiet, gentle way. Even light humor about the bizarreness of her situation may be appropriate. But be kind in your handling of the situation. The overriding principle is: Whatever you do, regard her feelings.

5. *Find things to praise her about.* Remember that depression is an illness of self-deprecation. During the illness, her self-esteem is at an all-time low. Don't criticize her; that adds to the bulk of evidence she is accumulating against herself. Find things to praise her about. Pay her

compliments. These should be sincere and not overdone flattery. She really does want to be capable and worthy of appreciation.

6. *Remove any obvious pressures and worries.* Your approach should be one of, "What can I do to help?" Be sensitive to your depressed friend's life and to what is exerting so much pressure on her. Then ask yourself, what can I do to help with any of those pressures?

I asked a woman who had been hospitalized twice for depression to come with me to a meeting where I was going to speak on depression. I felt she might benefit from the contact with the other women who would be there as well as gain some insights about her illness. Dana wanted to come, but didn't know what she would do with her children. I suggested she have her husband watch them. (Even finding a baby-sitter can seem like an impossible task to a depressed person.)

When Dana asked her husband, he said he had a golf game that afternoon and didn't want to have to hurry home to stay with the children. When Dana called to tell me what he had said, I quickly suggested someone else who might baby-sit. I couldn't understand her husband. Wasn't he concerned about his wife's illness? Why couldn't he quit playing golf a little earlier to help his wife?

The depressed woman sometimes feels like she is drowning in responsibilities. Everyone, she feels, is making exorbitant demands on her. If someone, friend or husband, can help with just one of those responsibilities, it can give her a burst of energy as well as lighten her load.

7. *Lighten the guilt.* No matter what caused a woman's depression, she is going to experience guilt with it. ("I shouldn't feel this way." Or, "I should be above this sort of thing.") Guilt is already present, so don't add to it. Don't make her feel bad because she is depressed. Depression may be a natural response to the stresses of life. Don't imply that if she were a capable woman or a mature Christian, she would not be depressed.

Neither should you make her feel guilt about taking antidepressant drugs, electroconvulsive treatment, or seeking professional help. These are legitimate forms of treatment. Be glad she is seeking help, and encourage her to continue to do so.

8. *Reassure her.* I found a contradiction in the material I read on helping people who are depressed. Some authorities said, "Reassure the depressed woman that her depression will end. Reassure her that things will get better. Over and over, she wants to hear that things will improve."

In contrast to that, other authorities said, "Don't convey the reassurance that she'll get over it or that things will get better. Things might not get better."

If it is a simple case of depression, you can take the advice of the first group of authorities. If a woman is suffering from depression after a move and she has not had any previous depressive episodes, you can reassure her that the depression will end. Given time, she will adjust to her new home and the depression will lift.

On the other hand, if it doesn't appear to be a simple case of depression, don't offer reassurance that it will end. Things may indeed get worse. I know. When Bob lost his job with the Christian university, one he felt God had called him to, some Christians said to me, "Oh, Bob will get another job. God's got something better for him." When he lost the next job, they were still saying the same thing. The advice was still the same when no church or college position was forthcoming. Their glib words sloughed off our pain and confusion.

Don't be guilty of offering cheap, unrealistic reassurance that ignores the depressed woman's pain or the seriousness of her situation. This is particularly difficult for Christians. Because we are people who walk by faith, we feel we must always be giving witness to that fact. If we can't offer solutions to people's problems, we feel like failures. We feel we must always state the truth and defend God. Job's friends were like that—so intent on defending God that they could not identify with Job. Job said to them, "You, however, smear me with lies; you are worthless physicians, all of you! If only you would be altogether silent! For you that would be wisdom" (Job 13:4, 5, NIV).

The kind of reassurance every depressed person needs is reassurance of your love. She needs to know that no matter what happens she is still a worthwhile person. "A pastor who had rather unskillfully (and fearfully) tried to help a woman through a depression-producing crisis by saying he was sure she would come out all right was told long afterward, 'What I most needed to know was not that I would come through all right, but that you and the others I respect would love me no matter what happened.' "[4]

9. *Plan interesting events.* Mobilization or a change of scene can break up the clutter of depressive thoughts. Depressed people often see no joy ahead, so Florence Littauer suggests planning an event ahead of time to give the depressed woman anticipation. "Men: think of something your wife would like to do and plan it. Don't ask if she wants to go away for a few days, just make the reservations. A change of scene can often give a new perspective to an old depression."[5]

Some couples can't afford to get away for a few days, so planning an event to anticipate may take some creative thinking on the part of the husband. Plan an evening out instead of a few days away. Hire a baby-sitter and plan where to go. Make it your idea and take care of all the details.

If an evening out is too expensive, then ask some friends to help you plan an "evening out" at home. Ask friends to take the children for an evening. Tell your wife you'll fix dinner *and* do the dishes. Plan simple food and serve it with candlelight. Think ahead of some questions you can ask your wife and then listen to her answers. Put on soft music. Getting her away from the house would be better; but an "evening out" at home can help relieve her too.

Women can do the same thing for their depressed friends.

Offer to buy your depressed co-worker lunch at a chic restaurant that's quiet. Or, have her over for brunch on Saturday morning. If she has children, then make plans for a baby-sitter. Take care of all the details, because stressful details can make a depressed woman feel the event is just not worth the trouble.

Encourage the depressed woman to do something with you, but don't force her. If she balks strongly, then leave her alone. Your offer will still be meaningful to her and show her that you care.

10. *Watch your own reaction.* Remember that depression is an illness that distorts a person's perspective and thinking patterns. The depressed person may do and say things that will make you angry and that sound utterly ridiculous. Be mad at the disease and not the person.

Depressives can be very convincing; even professional therapists have been convinced of the despair and hopelessness of certain patients. In your attempts to help, don't catch the illness in the sense that you, too, become depressed. Don't get discouraged.

Learn what you can about depression; be available; listen and try to understand; reassure her and plan interesting events. Then if she doesn't respond, don't feel guilty. "The depressed person is full of guilt and easily transfers this feeling to others. By their expressions and sighs they can make your conscience twinge. When you have done all you can to help the distressed person, rest in peace."[6] You are accountable to God for your actions, but not for another's reactions.

11. *Encourage her to get help.* The average length of a depressive illness is four months to one year. If a year has passed and your depressed friend is not better, then it is time to firmly and tactfully begin suggesting she get help. You will do her a tremendous favor if you will investigate the kinds of help available in your area. Find out the particulars and the cost. Share what you find with her. Offer to make an appointment for her and go with her.

If her thinking is severely distorted or she becomes incapable of handling her job or family, you may not want to wait a year. Encourage her to seek help immediately. You may need to be firm: "You are depressed. You need help. I know a doctor who can help. Let's go see him."

Encourage her to seek help because you love her. You want her to get well for her sake, not for yours. If she is your wife, don't say, "I wish you would get help for my sake or for the sake of the children. Think of us." If she is your friend, don't say, "You're killing our friendship by the way you are acting." Instead, a better approach is, "You are precious to me. I love you, and I want so much to see you feeling better."

12. *Treat any threat of suicide seriously.* A popular misconception is that people who talk about suicide don't commit it. That's not true; 80 percent of those who commit suicide give warnings of their intent to someone they know.

If your friend is seriously depressed, then be on the alert for signals of suicide intention. She may say something such as, "My husband will be sorry when I'm gone"; or, "I just can't go on feeling like this much longer"; or, "There's nothing left to live for." She may start putting business matters in order. Don't shrug off these symptoms. Instead, ask about her intentions.

"Don't be afraid to come right out and ask, 'Do you feel bad enough to kill yourself?' or 'Are you planning to kill yourself?' or 'Are you so upset that you are thinking of suicide?' "[7] This kind of questioning will not plant the idea of suicide in her mind. The idea is already there. Questioning will relieve her, giving her a chance to talk. The depressed woman, inwardly debating about committing suicide, is relieved to express her thoughts.

If she has a well-thought-out plan—naming time, place, and method—then she is past debating. She needs immediate help. Get her to a suicide prevention center, to a local mental health center, or to a doctor.

Your friend's intention of suicide is not something you

can handle alone. The depressed woman contemplating suicide needs professional help. In trying to help her, you can be alert to suicide signals and not brush them off; but don't take the responsibility of preventing her suicide by yourself.

The risk of suicide reminds us again that depression is an illness that may have devastating results. So if you care about the depressed woman in your life, you will reach out to her. Your faithful, listening presence may be the factor that will help preserve her life.

These twelve guidelines are given to help you know how to help her; but don't be worried about trying to conscientiously follow all twelve. Your availability and empathy are what matter most. These qualities will shine through whatever mistakes you may make.

Carileen (the woman to whom I dedicated this book) and I were casual acquaintances and fellow church members before my depressions. When Bob was fired the second time, she realized what a blow it was to me. She took me to lunch, and a friendship began. When Bob didn't get a church position and became an executive recruiter, she again sensed my disappointment and confusion. From then on, she frequently took me to lunch and kept in regular contact by phone. For a time, we haggled over God's purpose; she wanted so much to convince me that there was one. She'd present her side with a Scripture passage, and I would counter with another. There were times when I would get irritated with her, and I know there were many times when she lost her patience with me or thought I was overdoing it. As I look back, I don't recall a profound statement she made or a Scripture passage she quoted that ever made a difference in my depression. Her loyalty and her confidence in me as a person worth salvaging are what helped. I'll always be grateful to her for sensing my need and for standing by me.

One military wife who became depressed after too many moves too close together said a friend recognized the devastation she was experiencing. The friend regularly sent her verses of Scripture. The military wife said it wasn't actually what the verses said that helped her. It was having someone recognize what she was feeling and caring enough to do something about it on a continuing basis. What's important in helping a depressed woman is faithfulness, understanding her feelings, and recognizing her as a person of worth.

The depressed woman is groping in darkness—a darkness so thick that it even blocks the light of God from getting through. While God's light is temporarily blocked, she needs someone who has access to that light to walk through the darkness with her. You can be God's light to the woman in darkness.

[1]Fairchild, *op. cit.*, p. 56.
[2]Millard Osborne, "The Word of Loneliness," in *The Way of the Cross and Resurrection*, edited by John M. Drescher (Scottdale, Penn.: Herald Press, 1978), p. 157.
[3]Florence Littauer, *Blow Away the Black Clouds*, (Eugene, Ore.: Harvest House Publishers, 1979), p. 103.
[4]Fairchild, *op. cit.*, p. 75.
[5]Littauer, *op. cit.*, p. 104.
[6]*Ibid.*, pp. 104, 105.
[7]Fairchild, *op. cit.*, p. 97.

SELECTED BIBLIOGRAPHY

Barrett, Roger, *Depression—What It Is and What to Do About It*, Elgin, Illinois, David C. Cook Publishing Co., 1977.

Burns, David D., *Feeling Good: The New Mood Therapy*, New York, New York, William Morrow and Co., Inc., 1980.

Fairchild, Roy W., *Finding Hope Again: A Pastor's Guide to Counseling Depressed Persons*, San Francisco, California, Harper & Row Publishers, Inc., 1980.

LaHaye, Tim, *How to Win Over Depression*, Grand Rapids, Michigan, Zondervan Publishing House, 1974.

Littauer, Florence, *Blow Away the Black Clouds*, Eugene, Oregon, Harvest House Publishers, 1979.

Minirth, Frank B., and Meier, Paul D., *Happiness Is a Choice, a Manual on the Symptoms, Causes, and Cures of Depression*, Grand Rapids, Michigan, Baker Book House, 1978.

Osborne, Cecil, *The Art of Understanding Your Mate*, Grand Rapids, Michigan, Zondervan Publishing House, 1970.

Scarf, Maggie, *Unfinished Business: Pressure Points in the Lives of Women*, Garden City, New York, Doubleday, 1980.